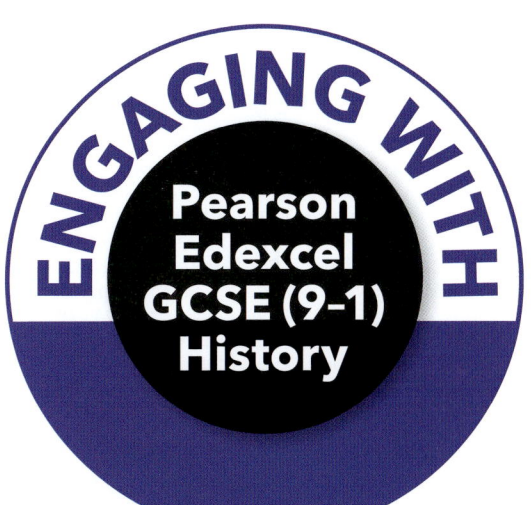

MEDICINE IN BRITAIN c1250–PRESENT

AND THE BRITISH SECTOR OF THE WESTERN FRONT, 1914–1918

SAM SLATER
DALE BANHAM

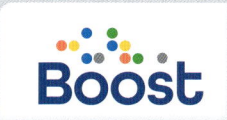
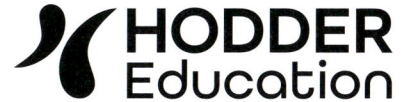

The Publishers would like to thank the following for permission to reproduce copyright material.

Photo credits

p.10tl © Photo Researchers/Science History Images/Alamy Stock Photo; **p.10bl** © Jochen Tack/ImageBROKER.com GmbH & Co. KG /Alamy Stock Photo; **p.10tr** © Wellcome Collection, London/http://creativecommons.org/licenses/by/4.0/; **p10.br** © Musée Condé, Chantilly/Bridgeman Images; **p.14** © Science History Images/Alamy Stock Photo; **p.17** © Marzolino/Shutterstock; **p.18t** © SHEILA TERRY/SCIENCE PHOTO LIBRARY; **p.18b** © From the British Library archive/Bridgeman Images; **p.20** © Attribution 4.0 International (CC BY 4.0) via Wellcome Collection; St. Bartholomew's Hospital, Mediaeval Period; **p.21** © Gianni Dagli Orti/Shutterstock; **p.22** © Attribution 4.0 International (CC BY 4.0) via Wellcome Collection; **p.14** Ms 89 fol.88 The Triumph of Death, from a Book of Hours (vellum), French School, (15th century) / ©Bibliotheque Municipale, Moulins, France / Bridgeman Images; **p.25** © The Print Collector / Alamy Stock Photo; **p.33** © GRANGER - Historical Picture Archive / Alamy Stock Photo; **p.34** © Wellcome Library, London. Wellcome Images/http://creativecommons.org/licenses/by/4.0/ **p.35t** © Printers working at a printing press, and setting type. Woodcut by J. Amman. Wellcome Collection. Public Domain Mark. Source: Wellcome Collection; **p.35b** © From the British Library archive/Bridgeman Images; **p.36** © Wellcome Collection, London/http://creativecommons.org/licenses/by/4.0/; **p.37** © The Book Worm/Alamy Stock Photo; **p.38t** © Classicpaintings/Alamy Stock Photo; **p.38b** © Wellcome Collection, London/http://creativecommons.org/licenses/by/4.0/; **p.40** © LAURA/stock.adobe.com; **p.43t** © Wellcome Collection.Public Domain Mark 1.0; **p.43b** © World History Archive / Alamy Stock Photo; **p.47** © Granger Historical Picture Archive / Alamy Stock Photo; **p.48** © Granger Historical Picture Archive / Alamy Stock Photo; **p.54** © Wellcome Collection.https://creativecommons.org/licenses/by/4.0/; **p.56** © Wellcome Images/ Attribution 4.0 International (CC BY 4.0); **p.59** © North Wind Picture Archives / Alamy Stock Photo; **p.60** © Wellcome Collection, London/http://creativecommons.org/licenses/by/4.0/; **p.62** © Wellcome Collection, London/http://creativecommons.org/licenses/by/4.0/; **p.63** © Pictorial Press Ltd / Alamy Stock Photo; **p.66** © Historic England Archive/Heritage Image Partnership Ltd/Alamy Stock Photo; **p.70** © Wellcome Library, London. Wellcome Images/http://creativecommons.org/licenses/by/4.0/; **p.71** © Wellcome Collection, London/http://creativecommons.org/licenses/by/4.0/; **p.75** © Wellcome Collection. https://creativecommons.org/licenses/by/4.0/; **p.76l** © Elizabeth Leyden/Alamy Stock Photo; **p.76r** © London Stereoscopic Company/Hulton Archive/Getty Images; **p.79t** © GL Archive / Alamy Stock Photo; **p.79b** © Wellcome Collection. https://creativecommons.org/licenses/by/4.0/; **p.82** © Keystone Press/Alamy Stock Photo; **p.84** © Hulton-Deutsch Collection/CORBIS/Getty Images; **p.87** A. BARRINGTON BROWN, © GONVILLE & CAIUS COLLEGE/COLOURED BY SCIENCE PHOTO LIBRARY; **p.89** Reproduced with the kind permission of Alcohol Change UK; **p.90** © Choja/E+/Getty Images; **p.91** © Image Supply Co/stock.adobe.com; **p.95** © Popperfoto/Getty Images; **p.96** © Science Museum, London. https://creativecommons.org/licenses/by/4.0/; **p.97** © Chronicle/Alamy Stock Photo; **p.98** © Lebrecht Music & Arts / Alamy Stock Photo; **p.99** © Manfred Weis/Westend61 GmbH/Alamy Stock Photo; **p.100** © Shawshots/Alamy Stock Photo; **p.101** © Pikselstock/stock.adobe.com; **p.102** © Bridgeman Images; **p. 107t** © Bloomsbury Academic, an imprint of Bloomsbury Publishing Plc; **p. 107br** Cover design by Simi Abe. Cover images from a series of portraits from The Allies by Eugene Burnand (1850-1921), (pencil and pastel on paper) © Birmingham Museums Trust **p.107bl** Courtesy of the British Association of Plastic, Reconstructive and Aesthetic Surgeons; **p.109t** © Wellcome Collection/ Attribution 4.0 International (Public domain mark 1.0); **p.109b** © Bettmann/Getty Images; **p.111** Image Courtesy of the National Army Museum, London; **p.113** © Shawshots/Alamy Stock Photo; **p.114** © Look and Learn/Bridgeman Images; **p.115** Image Courtesy of the National Army Museum, London; **p.117** © IWM Q 10622; **p.118l** © IWM HU 109801; **p.118r** © IWM Art.IWM ART 1460; **p.119** © IWM Q 1778; **p.121** © IWM Q 107977; **p.124** © IWM Q 10622; **p.128** © Science & Society Picture Library/Getty Images; **p.129** © Science & Society Picture Library/Getty Images; **p.132** © The National Archives

Although every effort has been made to ensure that website addresses are correct at time of going to press, Hodder Education cannot be held responsible for the content of any website mentioned in this book. It is sometimes possible to find a relocated web page by typing in the address of the home page for a website in the URL window of your browser.

Hachette UK's policy is to use papers that are natural, renewable and recyclable products and made from wood grown in well-managed forests and other controlled sources. The logging and manufacturing processes are expected to conform to the environmental regulations of the country of origin.

To order, please visit www.hoddereducation.com or contact Customer Service at education@hachette.co.uk / +44 (0)1235 827827.

ISBN: 9781398389229

© Sam Slater and Dale Banham 2024
First published in 2023 by Hodder Education,
An Hachette UK Company
Carmelite House
50 Victoria Embankment
London EC4Y 0DZ

www.hoddereducation.com

Impression number   10 9 8 7 6 5 4 3 2 1

Year   2028 2027 2026 2025 2024

All rights reserved. Apart from any use permitted under UK copyright law, no part of this publication may be reproduced or transmitted in any form or by any means, electronic or mechanical, including photocopying and recording, or held within any information storage and retrieval system, without permission in writing from the publisher or under licence from the Copyright Licensing Agency Limited. Further details of such licences (for reprographic reproduction) may be obtained from the Copyright Licensing Agency Limited, www.cla.co.uk

Cover photo © Historical image collection by Bildagentur-online / Alamy Stock Photo

Illustrations by Integra

Typeset in India

Printed and bound in Great Britain by Bell & Bain Ltd, Glasgow

A catalogue record for this title is available from the British Library.

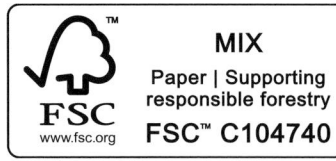
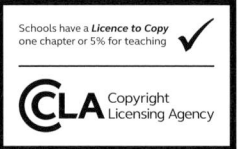

CONTENTS

Introduction to the thematic study 4

Part 1: c1250–c1500: Medicine in medieval England 14

Ideas about the cause of disease and illness c1250–c1500 14

Approaches to prevention and treatment c1250–c1500 17

Case study: Dealing with the Black Death, 1348–49 24

Medieval medicine period review 26

Part 2: c1500–c1700: The Medical Renaissance in England 30

Ideas about the cause of disease and illness c1500–1700 30

Approaches to prevention and treatment c1500–1700 36

Case study: William Harvey and the discovery of the circulation of the blood 42

Case study: Dealing with the Great Plague in London, 1665 46

Medical Renaissance period review 49

Part 3: c1700–c1900: Medicine in eighteenth- and nineteenth-century Britain 54

Ideas about the cause of disease and illness c1700–1900 54

Approaches to treatment c1700–1900 58

Approaches to prevention c1700–1900 70

Case study: Jenner and the development of vaccination 70

Case study: Fighting cholera in London, 1854 74

Eighteenth- and nineteenth-century medicine period review 80

Part 4: c1900–present: Medicine in modern Britain 82

Case study: Fleming, Florey and Chain's development of penicillin 82

Ideas about the cause of disease and illness c1900–present 86

Approaches to prevention and treatment c1900–present 92

Case study: The fight against lung cancer in the twenty-first century 102

Medicine in modern Britain period review 104

Part 5: The British sector of the Western Front, 1914–18: injuries, treatment and the trenches 106

How do we know about injuries and treatments in the British sector of the Western Front, 1914–18? 106

The historical context of medicine in the early twentieth century 108

The British sector of the Western Front 112

Conditions requiring medical treatment on the Western Front 116

Medical treatment on the Western Front 120

The significance of the Western Front for experiments in surgery and medicine 126

The British sector of the Western Front, 1914–18; injuries, treatment and the trenches period review 130

Glossary 134

Index 136

Introduction to the thematic study

0.1 Your exam: What is assessed and how

The GCSE course that you are following is made up of four different studies.

	Paper 1: Thematic study and historic environment	Paper 2: Period study and British depth study	Paper 3: Modern depth study
What is assessed?	**Section A: Historic environment** This focuses on the relationship between a place and historical events and developments. **Section B: Thematic study** This focuses on change and continuity across a long sweep of history – from the medieval period to the present day.	**Option P: Period study** This focuses on a wider world topic over a period of at least 50 years. **Option B: British depth study** This focuses on a period of British history over a shorter period of time (under 40 years).	This focuses on the complexity of a historical society or situation. The interplay of different aspects of history are considered.
How is it assessed?	Written exam: 1 hour 20 minutes 30% of your GCSE (52 marks) Section A – 3 compulsory questions (16 marks) Section B – 2 compulsory questions and 1 from a choice of 2 (36 marks)	Written exam: 1 hour 50 minutes 40% of your GCSE (64 marks) **Period study** – 2 compulsory questions and 2 from a choice of 3 (32 marks) **British depth study** – 2 compulsory questions and 1 from a choice of 2 (32 marks)	Written exam: 1 hour and 30 minutes 30% of your GCSE (52 marks) Section A – 1 compulsory question and one from a choice of 2 (16 marks) Section B – 4 compulsory questions (36 marks)

This book prepares you for Paper 1: Medicine in Britain, c1250–present and The British Sector of the Western Front, 1914–18: injuries, treatment and the trenches.

It focuses on how medicine developed in Britain over a long period of time. You will study:

- how key features in the development of medicine were linked with the key features of society in Britain across different time periods
- the causes and consequences of the developments that took place in medicine
- the significance of key developments, individuals and events
- the nature and process of change. This will involve understanding patterns of change, trends and turning points, and the influence of factors encouraging or inhibiting change within periods and across themes in medicine.

Period and theme	Key content	Period review pages
1 Medicine in medieval England, c1250–c1500 *Medicine stands still*	• Medieval ideas about the cause of disease and illness • Medieval approaches to prevention and treatment • Medical training and traditional approaches to treatment and care of the sick • Case study: Dealing with the Black Death, 1348–49	Pages 26–27

Period and theme	Key content	Period review pages
2 The Medical Renaissance in England, c1500–c1700 *The beginnings of change*	• The beginning of a scientific approach to the causes of disease and illness during the Medical Renaissance • Continuity and change in approaches to prevention, treatment and care • The impact of improvements in medical training • Case studies: William Harvey and the discovery of the circulation of the blood and Dealing with the Great Plague in London, 1665	Pages 49–50
3 Medicine in eighteenth- and nineteenth-century Britain, c1700–c1900 *A revolution in medicine*	• The influence in Britain of Pasteur's Germ Theory and Koch's work on microbes • Improvements in hospital care and the influence of Nightingale, Simpson and Lister • New approaches to the prevention of disease and illness • Case studies: Jenner and the development of vaccination and Fighting cholera in London, 1854	Pages 80–81
4 Medicine in modern Britain, c1900–present *Modern medicine*	• The influence of genetics and lifestyle factors on understanding the cause of disease and illness, and improvements in diagnosis • Changes in care and treatment because of the NHS and science and technology • New approaches to the prevention of disease and illness • Case studies: Fleming, Florey and Chain's development of penicillin and The fight against lung cancer in the twenty-first century	Pages 104–105
5 The British sector of the Western Front, 1914–18	• The significance of the terrain on the British sector of the Western Front on medical treatment • Conditions requiring treatment on the Western Front • Medical treatment on the Western Front • The significance of the Western Front for experiments in surgery and medicine	Pages 130–131

> ### Revision Tip
>
> **Break down your revision into manageable chunks of content**
>
> This book is organised into five parts that reflect the parts of the specification. At the end of each part of the course, make sure you review and revise what you have just covered. The 'Exam Practice', 'Recall Challenge' and 'Review' features will help you do this.

How the thematic study will be examined

> **Exam Tip**
>
> You should always spend up to 2 minutes making sure you identify the focus of the question and planning your approach before you start to write your answer.

Type of question		Guidance	Marks	Writing time	Advice and practice
Section A: The historic environment: The British sector of the Western Front, 1914–18: injuries, treatment and the trenches					
These questions require you to analyse and evaluate historical sources (contemporary to the period)					
1	Q1a: Describe one feature of … Q1b: Describe one feature of …	Focus on the question – identify a feature and then support with a sentence of historical information. Repeat for the second feature.	2 2	6 minutes	Pages 115, 117, 119, 121 and 132
2a	How useful are Sources A and B for an enquiry into …	The sources could be visual or written. They will relate to an aspect of the enquiry in the question. Focus on how the sources are useful. Use the content of the sources, the provenance of the sources and your contextual knowledge to evaluate the usefulness of the sources.	8	12 minutes	Pages 115, 124–125 and 132–133
2b	How could you follow up Source A/B to find out more about …	Identify a detail from the content of the source linked to the enquiry in the question. Write a question that will provide you with more information for the enquiry. Identify a contemporary source and make it specific to the enquiry. Check that it will have the answer to your question. Explain how the source will answer your question.	4	6 minutes	Pages 125 and 132–133

Type of question		Guidance	Marks	Writing time	Advice and practice
Section B: Thematic study: Medicine in Britain, c1250–present These questions focus on second order concepts such as continuity, change, cause, consequence, significance, similarity and difference.					
3	Explain one way … similar/different …	Focus on the question – explain a similarity or difference. Support with historical examples from both time periods in the question.	4	6 minutes	Pages 39, 41, 50, 68, 81, 89, 97, 103 and 105
4	Explain why ….	Focus on the question – explain why there was change in medicine. Aim to write three paragraphs. Support your answer with at least three aspects of knowledge.	12	18 minutes	Pages 19, 44–45, 68–69, 73, 85, 99 and 105
5/6	'Statement': How far do you agree?	This is an essay question, requiring you to reach a judgement. Aim to agree with the statement and then disagree with an alternative argument. Support your answer with at least three aspects of knowledge. Make sure that you write a conclusion explaining how far you agree with the statement.	20 (16 + 4 for SPAG)	27 minutes	Pages 28–29, 33, 51–53, 81 and 105

Revision Tips

Make exam practice part of your revision

Exam Tips give you step-by-step guidance on how to tackle each type of question. Effective revision is not just learning the content. You need to understand what each type of question is asking you to think about in the exam and to practise delivering it.

Take responsibility

Reflect on your strengths and weaknesses. What question types do you struggle with? Take responsibility: spend more time practising the types of question you find most difficult. Use feedback from your teacher to improve your approach.

0.2 The Big Picture: Identify the key questions

Connect & Engage

The period summaries below identify people and events that have shaped medicine in Britain since c1250. They also show the big questions you will cover. However, top history students do not only answer other people's questions, they also ask questions of their own!

As you read each summary, note down your own questions (large or small) about each period.

PART 1: c1250–c1500: Medicine in medieval England *Medicine stands still*

Big question: Why did medicine change so little in medieval England?

Ideas about the cause of disease and illness	Methods of prevention and treatment
• Some medieval people believed God sent illness to punish people for their sins. Others believed that people who became ill had breathed in bad air. • Specialist doctors called **physicians** treated the rich. • In the 1200s, universities were set up and physicians were trained there. They read the works of **Galen** (a doctor from Ancient Rome). • Galen blamed sickness on the four **humours** (liquids) in the body being out of balance.	• Most medieval people would pray to God for forgiveness and healing. • If a sick person went to a physician, he checked their urine to see if their humours were out of balance. He balanced them by **bleeding** (taking blood from the body) or **purging** (making the person vomit). • Most people could not afford to see a physician. They were treated at home or by the local wise woman with **herbal remedies**. • Hospitals were set up and run by the Church. They provided prayer, rest and food, not medical treatments. • When a terribly bad outbreak of **plague** called the **Black Death** arrived in 1348, it killed around 40 per cent of the population. People could not treat the victims or stop the plague spreading.

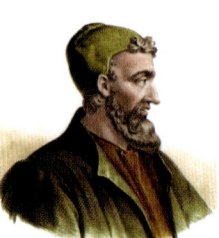

PART 2: c1500–c1700: The Medical Renaissance England *The beginnings of change*

Big question: How far were the ideas of Hippocrates and Galen challenged during the Renaissance?

Ideas about the cause of disease and illness	Methods of prevention and treatment
• Most people continued to believe that God or bad air or unbalanced humours made people sick. • **Andreas Vesalius** improved knowledge of anatomy (the structure of the body) by dissecting dead bodies. • **William Harvey** discovered that blood circulates round the body. • **Thomas Sydenham** encouraged doctors to closely observe their patients when diagnosing disease and illness. • Knowledge spread more quickly because of the invention of the printing press and The Royal Society.	• Vesalius and Harvey improved medical knowledge, but they did not cure illnesses. Prayer and herbal remedies remained common treatments. Physicians still used bleeding and purging to balance humours. • There were more hospitals and they started to provide specialised care (for example, maternity wards). • There was a serious outbreak of plague in London in 1665 but, just like in 1348, no one could stop it.

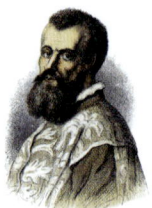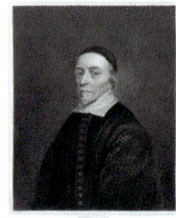

PART 3: c1700–c1900: Medicine in eighteenth- and nineteenth-century Britain
A revolution in medicine

Big question: How did the Germ Theory revolutionise medicine?

Ideas about the cause of disease and illness

- In 1861, **Louis Pasteur** published his **Germ Theory** which showed that bacteria (**germs**) cause diseases. He carried out experiments to prove his theory was correct.
- However, some people still believed that bad air caused illness because diseases spread most rapidly in the dirtiest, smelliest industrial towns.

Methods of prevention and treatment

- In the 1700s, there was growing interest in scientific medicine and old ideas were challenged. New methods of treatment were tried out, for example **Edward Jenner** invented **vaccination** to prevent people catching smallpox.
- Pasteur's theory led to preventions for killer diseases.
- Germ Theory also led to the development of **antiseptics** to prevent infection during surgery and helped persuade governments to pass laws to improve **public health**.
- Surgery was also improved by better scientific knowledge (particularly in chemistry) and the development of anaesthetics that prevented patients from suffering pain during operations.
- Meanwhile, improvements in engineering helped to provide the sewer systems that would clean up the growing towns and cities during the Industrial Revolution.
- Not everything changed. People still used herbal remedies, some of which did help the sick.

PART 4: c1900–present: Medicine in modern Britain *Modern medicine*

Big question: How has the government's role in medicine changed since c1900?

Ideas about the cause of disease and illness

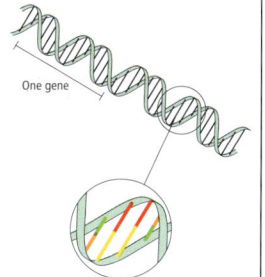

- In the 1950s, scientists discovered the existence of **DNA**, the 'building blocks' of the human body. This led to much more research which identified the individual **genes** that cause some illnesses.
- It is now understood that people's lifestyle can cause disease and illness.

Methods of prevention and treatment

- Developments in science and technology greatly improved surgery, for example by identifying blood groups which made blood **transfusions** effective.
- The discovery and development of chemical drugs and then **antibiotics** in the 1940s saved millions of lives by providing cures for illnesses and infections.
- Wars forced governments to invest more in improving public health. During the twentieth century, governments introduced better education, housing and public health provision.
- In 1942, the **Beveridge Report** (produced by **William Beveridge**) created the plan for the National Health Service (**NHS**), which began in 1948. For the first time, the NHS provided everyone with free treatment from a doctor at the point of delivery, so they were more likely to get help before an illness became serious.

PART 5: The British sector of the Western Front, 1914–18: injuries, treatment and the trenches

Big question: What can we learn from sources about the injuries, treatment and the trenches at the British sector of the Western Front?

- The terrain and conditions in the trenches led to illness and injuries for the soldiers, including trench foot and head injuries.
- The use of gas led to new injuries and treatment.
- A system of transporting the wounded was developed to overcome the problems caused by the terrain and trench warfare.
- Experiments in surgery and medicine took place leading to new techniques in the treatment of wounds and infection including the Thomas Splint and the creation of a blood bank.

0.3 Factors that help to explain change and continuity in medicine

Research & Record

What factors influenced the history of medicine?

We are incredibly lucky to be living now and not 500 or even 100 years ago. As Graph 1 shows, we live far longer than our ancestors. We are healthier and have a greater chance of surviving major illnesses.

So, why has medicine changed so much in recent times? That's what this course is all about. The cards on page 11 show the main factors that have affected medicine and health.

1. Pictures A–D show people being treated during different periods. Which time period does each image show?

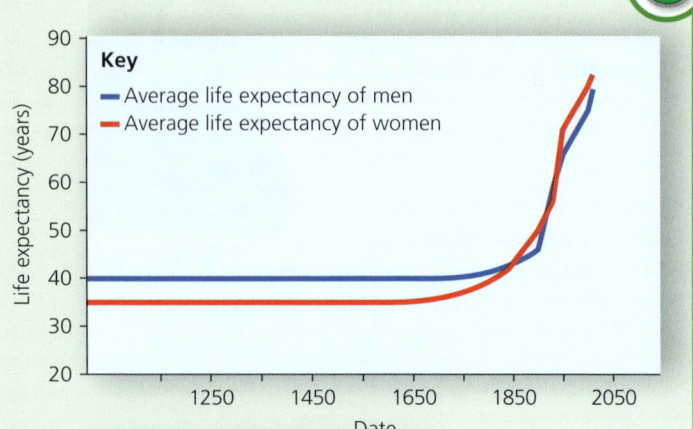
▲ Graph 1

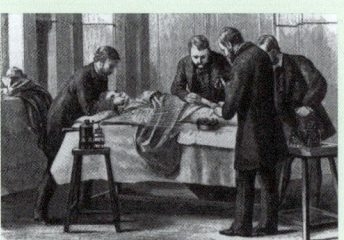
▲ Picture A

2. Can you match one factor from page 11 to each picture?

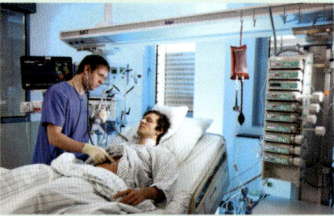
▲ Picture B

3. Look back at the Big Picture on pages 8–9. What factors can you see influencing medicine and health in each period?

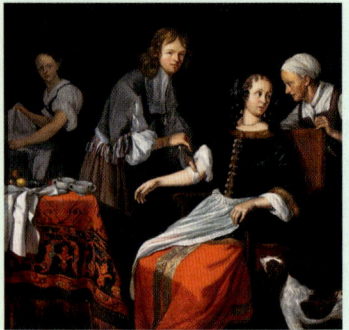
▲ Picture C

4. Make a large copy of a table like the one below to record your research. Keep this table and add to it throughout your course. Make sure you provide evidence to support your answers.

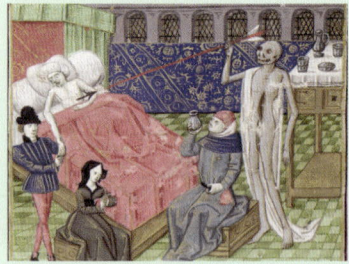
▲ Picture D

Period	Factors that influenced developments	Evidence
Medicine stands still (c1250–c1500)	The Church	Hospitals were set up and run by the Church
The beginnings of change (c1500–c1700)		
A revolution in medicine (c1700–c1900)		
Modern medicine (c1900–present)		

Throughout this course, you need to look for change and continuity in medicine in Britain. Consider when change or continuity took place. Consider why medicine changed or continued. Begin to reach judgements about how much change and continuity took place.

Change
When the ideas about the cause of disease and illness and approaches to prevention and treatment were different from previously.

Continuity
When ideas about the cause of disease and illness and approaches to prevention and treatment stayed the same as previously.

The role of individuals
Individuals have greatly influenced medicine and public health. For example, during the Renaissance, individuals such as Vesalius and Harvey increased knowledge of how the body is structured (**anatomy**) and the way that it works (**physiology**).

The role of the Church
The Church has both encouraged and inhibited change. For example, in the medieval period, the Church set up hospitals and encouraged people to care for the sick. However, in medieval England, the Church also discouraged people from challenging old ideas and developing new ones.

The role of government
In modern medicine, government plays a crucial role. During the nineteenth century, it passed laws to force local town councils to provide clean water for people. Since the creation of the NHS in the 1940s, the government uses a large part of the taxes it collects to fund the service and to pay for medical research and vaccination programmes.

Science and technology
Developments in science and technological improvements have transformed medicine in the last 200 years. New inventions and equipment, such as X-ray machines, body scanners and lasers, have revolutionised the way that illness is diagnosed and treated.

Attitudes in society
Attitudes in society have both encouraged and inhibited change. For example, in the medieval period, people believed in the ideas of Galen and did not consider that he could be wrong. However, this changed in Renaissance England when people took a more scientific approach and carried out experiments to challenge the ideas of Galen.

Revision Tip
Take responsibility
Questions 4, 5 and 6 in the exam will test your knowledge and understanding of change and continuity in medicine in Britain. You can use the factors on this page to explain why there was change and continuity. These questions carry a lot of marks and the more care you give to completing the table on page 10, the better able you will be to write good answers.

0.4 Key features: How this book works

The tasks in this book will help you learn what you need to know and how to apply your knowledge to answer exam questions effectively. They are your **'steps to success'**.

Research & Record

This gets your learning into your head in the first place and into your notebook. It will start you thinking in a way that will help you produce good answers to the exam questions.

Each **research question** reflects an issue that examiners will expect you to be an expert on. Complete these tasks, which build an answer to each research question, carefully and neatly because they will become your revision notes. Many tasks use tables. Give yourself room – each table should have its own page in your notebook.

? If you have gaps in your knowledge, go back to your research notes and the relevant section of this book and make sure that you add anything that is missing so you have covered all the key topics in enough detail.

Summarise

This turns your learning into a **memorable form**. Sometimes we guide you to do this, but mostly it is up to you.

Memory aids are different from your research notes. They use images or diagrams but few words. Most people remember better if something is summarised with both text and visuals.

? If you cannot remember some of the content you have covered, go back to your research notes and improve or recreate your memory aid.

Connect & Engage

These tasks make you form **connections** between what you have already learned and what you are about to learn.

Apply ▶ Recall Challenge

Prepare yourself for exams by testing yourself on what you have learned.

Quizzes, games and competitions test how much you can remember. They identify your weak spots where you need to spend more time.

Apply ▶ Exam Practice

Continue to prepare for the exam by answering exam-style questions with our Exam Tips to guide you.

Our **practice questions** are like the questions you will be asked in the exam, although none come from actual past papers. You can get real papers from your teacher or the Edexcel website. There are **Exam Tips** for each question type so you know how to approach them.

? If you did not understand how to approach an exam question, go back to the Exam Tips in this book and re-read them, checking that you fully understand what is required in a good answer to that type of question.

Review

We regularly **review** the **big ideas and concepts**. We also encourage you to **review your own learning**.

? **Take responsibility**
Review your own learning. What areas did you do well on? What areas do you need to improve?

Revision Tips

1. **Don't delay** revision until just before the exam. Revision should be an ongoing process. You need to revisit topics that you have studied regularly. Otherwise, as the graph shows, you will quickly start to forget key topics.
2. **Retrieval practice** makes your memory stronger. When you recall what you have previously studied, your brain strengthens connections and makes it easier to recall this information in the future.
3. **Spaced practice** helps you remember for longer! At the end of each topic, we test you, not just on that topic but on previous ones as well. You should regularly return to the Review tasks from previous topics and test your knowledge of 'older material'. As the graph shows, this should improve recall and stop you forgetting.

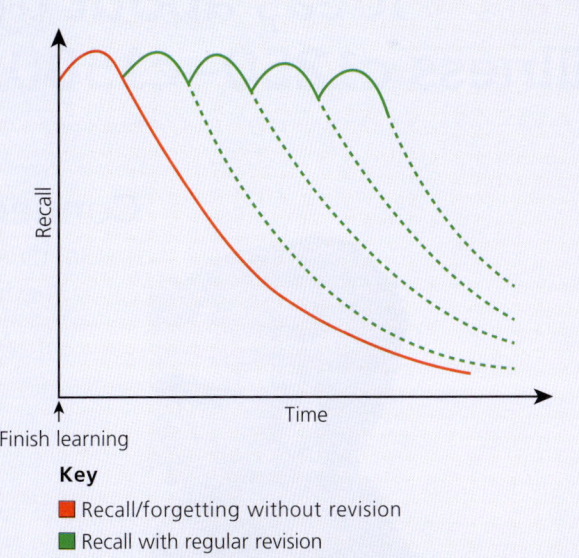

Key
- Recall/forgetting without revision
- Recall with regular revision

Apply ▶ Recall Challenges

1 Know the key individuals

Match each person below with the correct description.

Key individual	How their work influenced the development of medicine
Galen	Developed a vaccination against smallpox
Vesalius	Developed the Germ Theory
Harvey	Wrote a report recommending the setting up of the National Health Service
Sydenham	Described how the heart acts as a pump and circulates blood around the body
Jenner	A Roman doctor whose books influenced medicine in the medieval and Renaissance periods
Pasteur	Produced a book called *On the Fabric of the Human Body* which accurately described the structure of the body (anatomy)
Beveridge	Improved diagnosis of disease and illness during the Renaissance period

2 Know the key words

Match each key word below with its definition or description.

Key words	Definition/description
Antibiotics	An event that killed nearly half the population of England during the Middle Ages
Antiseptics	A belief that people became ill because liquids in the body were out of balance
Anaesthetics	The injection into the body of killed or weakened organisms to give the body resistance against the disease
The NHS	Chemicals used to destroy bacteria and prevent infection
The four humours	A group of drugs used to treat and cure infections caused by bacteria
The Black Death	A drug given to produce unconsciousness before and during surgery
Vaccinations	Set up in 1948 to provide free healthcare to everyone at the point of delivery

Part 1 Ideas about the cause of disease and illness c1250–c1500

Connect & Engage – Claudius Galen

Claudius Galen was born in Greece in AD129 and began studying medicine when he was just 16 years old.

At the age of 20, he moved to Rome where he soon made a reputation for himself as a doctor. He became doctor for the Roman Emperor and his family.

The squealing pig

Galen was a great showman. He would do public 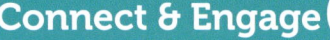 of animals and give talks.

In one famous performance, Galen showed his discoveries about the nervous system by dissecting a pig. As the pig squealed on the table, he cut into its neck, finding the nerves.

He could have cut through the correct nerve to stop the pig squealing immediately, but that did not appeal to Galen's showmanship. Instead, he announced, 'I will cut this nerve but the pig will keep squealing.' He cut, and the pig kept squealing. He cut again, building up the tension, and again the pig kept squealing.

Finally, he announced, 'When I cut this nerve, the pig will stop squealing.' He cut and the pig was silent!

Books, books and more books

Galen wrote over 300 books which covered every aspect of medicine. These were extremely detailed and well organised. They combined old Greek ideas (for example, the Theory of the Four Humours) with what he had learned from his own work.

Galen seemed to have covered everything so thoroughly that people believed his books contained all the answers. They became the basis for medical training for the next 1500 years.

People in the Middle Ages respected traditional ideas, so few tried to suggest alternative theories about what caused disease or how to treat it.

The support of the Church

One key reason Galen's books lasted so long was that his ideas fitted in with the ideas of the Christian Church, which controlled education in Europe in the Middle Ages.

Galen was not a Christian, but he taught that the body had been created by one god, who had made all the parts of the body fit together perfectly. This matched the Christian belief that God had created human beings.

Connect & Engage

Why did a doctor from Roman times still influence doctors 1500 years later?

1. List at least three reasons why Galen's work still influenced doctors in the Middle Ages.
2. Identify which of the following areas of medicine Galen influenced:
   A Ideas about the cause of disease
   B Approaches to prevention
   C Approaches to treatment

What were the key features of the ideas of Galen?

Galen's old ideas

- Galen also believed that people became sick when their humours were out of balance.
- He also recommended exercise and a good diet to stay healthy.
- His most common treatments were **bleeding** or making people vomit to restore the balance of the humours.

Galen's new ideas

The Theory of Opposites: Galen developed the idea of using 'opposites' to balance the humours. For example, if a patient had too much phlegm, then the illness was caused by cold. Galen's treatment was the opposite – he gave the patient a hot food such as peppers. This theory was popular because it was detailed and could be used to explain most illnesses. Doctors often fitted the symptoms they saw in a patient to the theory.

Dissection and knowledge of the body: Galen believed that physicians (doctors) should find out as much as possible about the anatomy of the body. He said that they should dissect human bodies themselves if they could and, if this was not possible, they should dissect apes because they were most like humans.

But... LIMITATIONS

Galen made mistakes because the bodies of apes and pigs are not the same as humans. Some of his mistakes went unchallenged for over a thousand years.

Long-term significance (the next 1500 years)

Because he wrote such good books, and had the support of the Church, doctors followed Galen's ideas for the next 1500 years. The Church made copies of Galen's books in monasteries, Church libraries always had copies of them, and Galen's books were used in Church medical schools.

Dissection was not allowed because the Church argued that the body needed to be buried whole for the soul to go to heaven. This meant that the ideas of Galen were not challenged.

The Theory of the Four Humours

This theory taught that:

- The body contains four humours or liquids (blood, phlegm, yellow bile and black bile).
- People became sick because they had too much or too little of one humour.
- For good health, humours needed to be balanced, so doctors gave advice on what to eat (diet) and how to exercise to stay in balance. They also bled patients or made them vomit to restore balance.
- People followed this theory because it made sense of the symptoms they observed. For example, a sick person might vomit yellow bile, or sneeze phlegm or bleed from the nose. This suggested that the body was unbalanced and was trying to get rid of too much of one humour.
- They also followed it because the advice on diet and exercise did work. Nowadays, we know that a balanced diet and exercise make you healthier. It was the same then.

Revision Tip

Create tables to summarise the ideas and approaches within each period. Start with the ideas of Galen. Look for these ideas as you learn about medicine in medieval England.

	Galen
Ideas about the cause of disease and illness	
Approaches to prevention and treatment	

Supernatural, religious and rational explanations of the cause of disease

> ### Research & Record
>
>
> **What were the ideas about the cause of disease and illness in medieval England?**
>
> Use this page to complete your own copy of a table like this. Record details of the **supernatural** and religious explanations (based on something that cannot be explained by nature) and the rational explanations (based on nature and logic).
>
> | Supernatural and religious explanations | Rational explanations |
> |---|---|
> | | |

A punishment from God

People looked to the Church to explain to them why terrible things happened. The most common belief was that God sent illnesses to punish people for their sins. To most people, this made sense, as they believed God created and controlled the world.

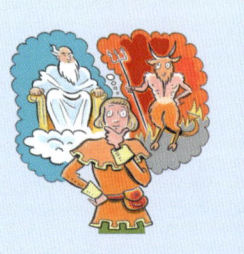

The Miasma Theory

A common explanation was that bad air filled with harmful smells was the cause of illness. This was called Miasma Theory. Some people linked the bad air to the filth in the streets but could not explain what the link was. This filth was caused by the poor systems of removing waste, including waste from butchers and animal dung.

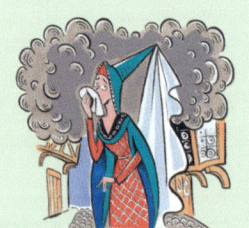

Astrology

Illness was sometimes linked to the movement of the planets and **astrology**. A physician would use the timing of a patient's birth and illness to consult star charts to decide what was wrong. People believed God controlled the planets and so gave more importance to this idea.

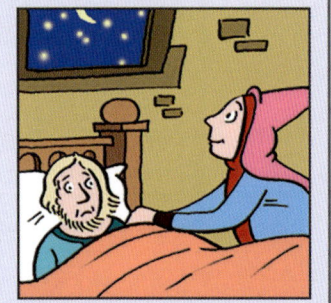

Theory of the Four Humours

Galen taught that people got ill when their humours were out of balance. Physicians had been trained using Galen's books, so they believed the same.

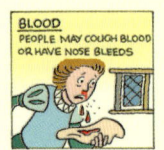 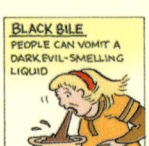 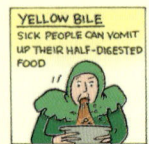 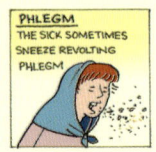

Part 1 Approaches to prevention and treatment c1250–c1500

Treating and preventing disease in medieval England

> ### Research & Record
>
> **How did ideas about the cause of disease and illness influence approaches to prevention and treatment?**
>
> Use pages 17–19 to complete your own copy of a table like this. Record examples of prevention and treatment linked to the main ideas.
>
> | Ideas about cause | Approaches to prevention and treatment |
> |---|---|
> | A punishment from God | |
> | Miasma Theory | |
> | Astrology | |
> | Theory of the Four Humours | |
> | Other | |

Religious actions

The Church taught that disease and illness was sent as a punishment from God for sin. As a result, people looked for religious treatments. This included prayer, fasting (going without food), and pilgrimages (journeys) to places of religious importance such as a shrine or a cathedral.

It was believed that the monarch had the power to heal certain illnesses. According to the theory of Divine Right, the king or queen was God's chosen representative on Earth, and it was believed that God had given them these powers. The monarch's touch was believed to cure scrofula, a skin disease.

Most people believed that the best way to prevent disease and illness was to lead a life free from sin. People were encouraged to attend church for prayer and confession.

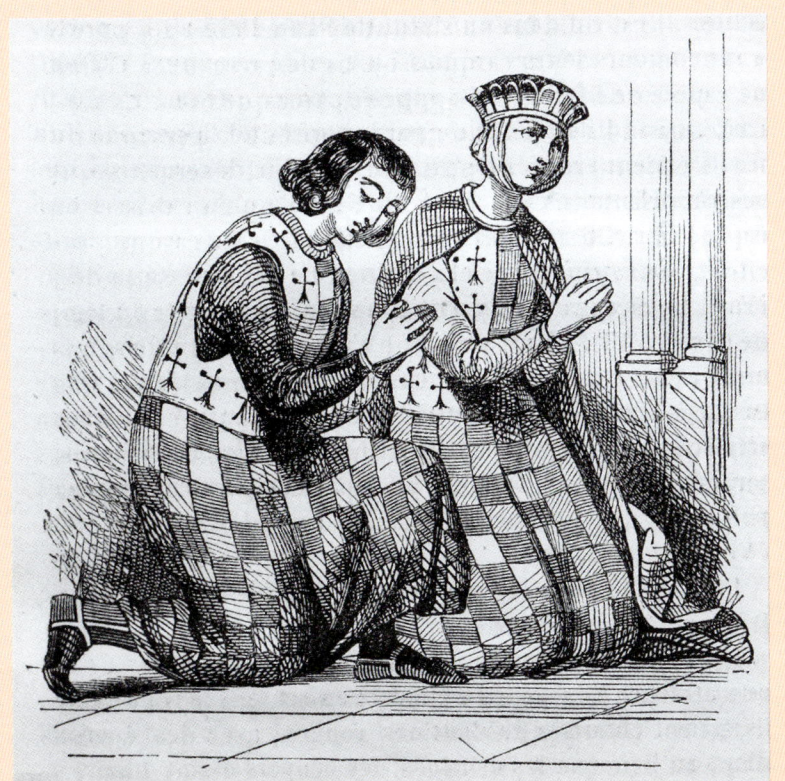

▲ **SOURCE A** Illustration of medieval prayer, drawn in the nineteenth century

Astrology

As well as being used for diagnosis, star charts were also used by physicians to prescribe treatment. The alignment of the planets was checked at every stage of the treatment, such as gathering herbs, bleeding the patient and operations. Every action had to happen at the correct time according to the stars.

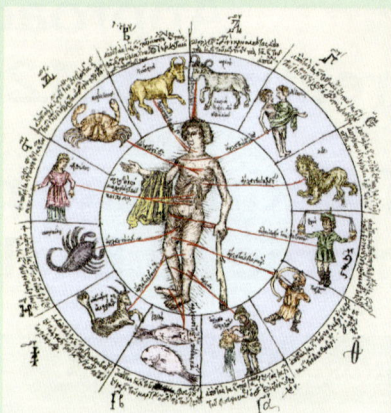

▲ **SOURCE B** A zodiac (star) chart from the fifteenth century

Bloodletting and purging

Bloodletting, or bleeding, was the most common treatment for an imbalance in the four humours. It was believed that removing blood also removed bad humours from the body. Bleeding of a patient took place by cutting a vein and placing leeches on the patient's skin, or placing heated cups over a cut or scratch to draw blood from the patient. These treatments were usually performed by a **barber surgeon**.

It was believed that the humours were created by the food a person ate. As a result, **purging** (removing any leftover food from the digestive system) was used as a treatment to balance the humours. This was achieved by giving the patient something to make them vomit or a laxative to clear out their bowels.

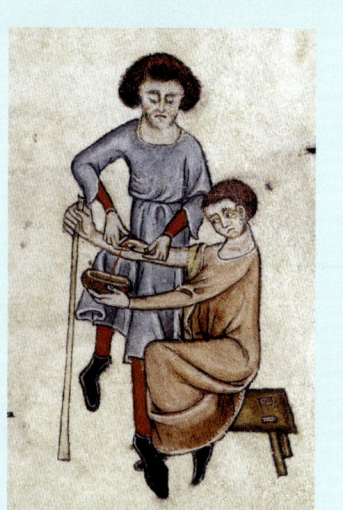

▲ **SOURCE C** An image from the Luttrel Psalter, a formal written document where the text is decorated with illustrations

Purifying the air

Medieval people would use many methods to keep the air clean and free from **miasma**. These included:
- carrying sweet-smelling herbs, such as lavender
- measures to keep the towns clean, such as removing any rotting animals from the streets, employing rakers to clean the streets, passing laws to punish people who threw their waste onto the streets, and building wells to provide fresh water.

Hygiene and diet

People believed that it was important to keep their body healthy to prevent illness and disease. Instructions for how to do this were written in the *Regimen Sanitatis*. People were advised to exercise, not to overeat, and keep clean by bathing. People could pay to visit a public bath or wash themselves in rivers to stay clean.

Exam Tip

Use connectives and evidence for stronger arguments

When explaining approaches to prevention and treatment in medicine, you have to prove the reason you have chosen was a cause in relation to the question. For example:

In medieval England, people believed religious actions would prevent and treat disease and illness. The Church was very influential, and many people believed that God sent disease and illness as a punishment for sin. **This led to** people using religious actions to prevent and treat disease and illness. **For example**, some people would use prayer and fasting. Other people would go on pilgrimages to visit religious places and holy shrines in the hope that God would forgive their sins and not send disease and illness. **This demonstrates** the important role that religion and the Church played in the approaches to prevention and treatment of disease and illness in medieval England.

Use connectives to tie what you know to the question

Phrases like 'this meant that', 'this led to' and 'this resulted in' are called connectives because they tie what you know to the question and so help you prove your argument.

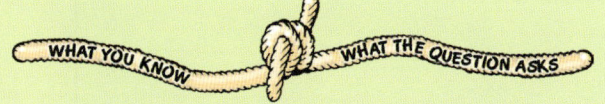

Add specific knowledge

Provide evidence to substantiate (support) your argument. Use phrases such as 'for example', 'such as' and 'this demonstrates' to introduce or flag your supporting evidence.

Apply ▶ Exam Practice

Question 4 style

Use the Exam Tip to complete two developed explanations.

1 The first explanation should prove that the Theory of the Four Humours led to preventions and treatments. You can base this on what you have read on these three pages.

2 The second explanation should prove that a belief in the Miasma Theory led to preventions.

Medical training and traditional approaches to treatment and care for the sick

> **Research & Record**
>
> **What care and treatment was provided in medieval hospitals?**
>
> Hospital care developed in medieval England as the number of hospitals increased.
>
> Use the information on this page to gather examples under both headings.
>
> | Treatment | Care |
> |---|---|
> | · Prayers | · Food |
> | · | · |
> | · | · |

Hospitals

The Christian Church taught that people should be looked after. This influenced the development of hospitals which appeared in towns throughout medieval England. One of the most famous was St Bartholomew's Hospital in London. The role of hospitals was to care for those who could no longer care for themselves, such as the poor and older people. Those with **infectious** illnesses were rarely admitted because they could spread the infection.

Hospitals were run by the Church. Monks and nuns provided food and drink, warmth and prayers. Nuns would also provide herbal treatments. The role of hospitals was 'care not cure' of the patients.

From the thirteenth century, smaller hospitals were founded. These were funded by wealthy townspeople to look after the citizens. By 1500, there were over 1000 hospitals in England. Some of these were specialist hospitals. In London, Richard Whittington, the Lord Mayor, paid for an eight-bed hospital for unmarried pregnant women. Leper houses were built outside towns to separate victims of **leprosy** from healthy people.

> **Connect & Engage**
>
> 1. What treatments can you see in Source E?
> 2. What evidence of care can you see in Source E?

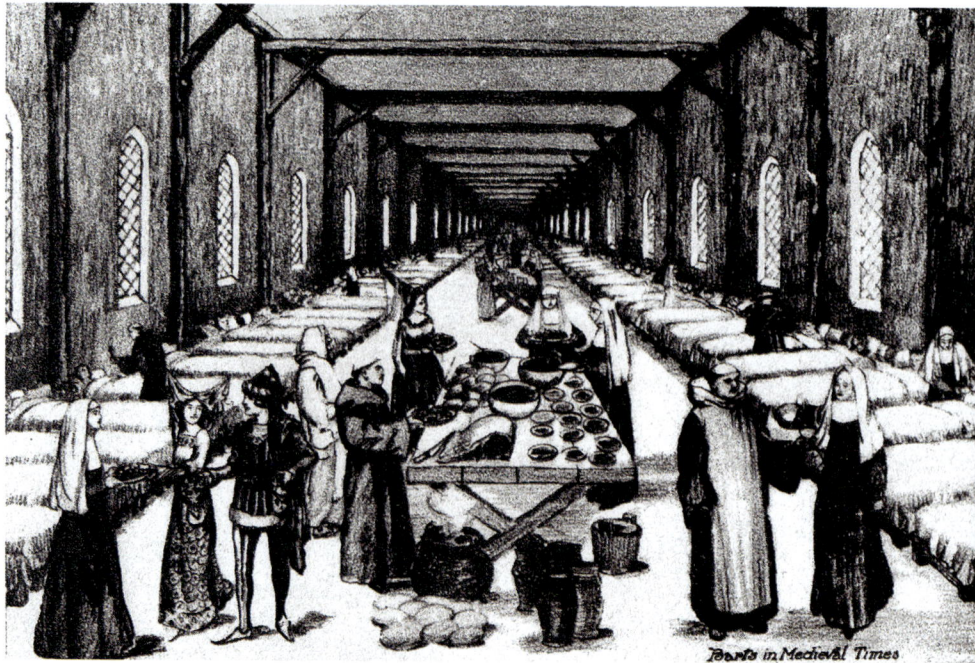

▶ **SOURCE D** An artist's impression of the inside of St Bartholomew's Hospital in the medieval period

The role of the physician, apothecary and barber surgeon in treatment and care

> **Research & Record**
>
> **Who treated and cared for the sick in medieval England?**
>
> Use the information on pages 20–21 to make notes about:
> - who treated and cared for the sick in medieval England
> - how they were trained
> - what treatments they provided.

Physician

Physicians were the highest-ranking doctors. They were well-paid. Only the rich could afford to go to a physician. They treated kings, nobles and wealthy merchants.

There were very few physicians. In the 1300s, there were less than 100 physicians in England. Women were not allowed to become physicians.

Treatments

The main role of a physician was to diagnose illness and advise a treatment. A physician would diagnose illness using the patient's urine, consulting a star chart, and by considering the balance of the patient's four humours.

Physicians advised on a range of treatments based on the Theory of the Four Humours. As well as bleeding or purging, they would advise patients how to stay healthy by regular washing, cleaning teeth, combing hair, exercising in the fresh air and bathing in hot water.

Training

Physicians were trained at university for seven years. They would have read the books written by Galen. The training was so expensive that only the rich could afford to enter this profession.

Source D shows one part of a physician's training – watching a dissection.

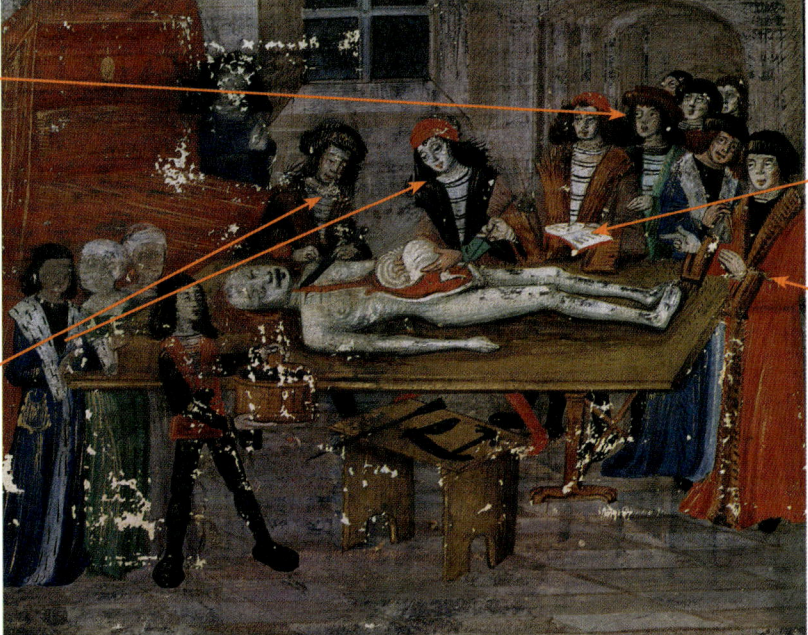

▲ **SOURCE E** A medieval painting showing part of the training for medieval doctors

Labels:
- Students – watching and listening
- Surgeons – doing the dissection
- Assistant – reading Galen's book out loud
- Physician – in charge

The physician (on the right) was in charge but did not do the dissection. He told the surgeon which part of the body to dissect. He also told his assistant (middle right) which passages of Galen to read out to illustrate the dissection. The students had to listen to Galen's words and watch the dissection. They were not allowed to do anything!

The dissections were designed to show that Galen's descriptions of the body were correct. They were not investigations to make new discoveries. Physicians believed that Galen's books contained everything they needed to learn about the human body.

Apothecary

Apothecaries were considered less knowledgeable than physicians. They were cheaper than a physician and so people would ask for their help as an alternative.

Treatments

Apothecaries made the herbal remedies. They mixed the ingredients to make the medicines for the physician.

Training

Apothecaries did not need to have attended university to set up their business. They would learn how to mix different remedies from other apothecaries or from family members.

Barber surgeon

Many medieval towns had a barber surgeon. They carried out treatments advised by physicians, or patients approached them directly if they could not afford to see a physician.

Treatments

Barber surgeons performed basic surgery such as bleeding, removing growths and tumours, and sewing up wounds. Occasionally, they would have to **amputate** a limb without an **anaesthetic** and so it was important that they had a steady hand.

Training

Barber surgeons were the least qualified medical professionals and were trained by watching others as an apprentice. They did not go to university. Women could become barber surgeons by working as an apprentice. Barber surgeons would get better with practice!

Women

Most people could not afford a physician, so they were treated at home by a member of their family – usually a woman.

Most women learned a wide range of remedies from their mother or grandmother, and they used these to treat their husbands and children. There might also be a wise woman in the village who they could consult when they did not know how to treat an illness.

These remedies were not just based on **superstition**. They sometimes worked.

Women also acted as midwives. In some towns, midwives had to serve an apprenticeship to learn the 'trade' and gain a licence to practise and were then paid for their expertise.

Use of remedies

Herbal remedies were also used to treat sick people in medieval England. These were usually given in the form of a herbal infusion that the patient would drink, inhale or bathe in. Common herbal remedies included aloe vera, camomile, rose oils and mint. Honey was often used in treatments for cuts and wounds. Today we know that this helped because it contains ingredients that fight infection. Different foods were recommended to balance out the humours.

Herbal remedies were recorded in books called 'herbals'. These included prayers to say while collecting and mixing the herbs.

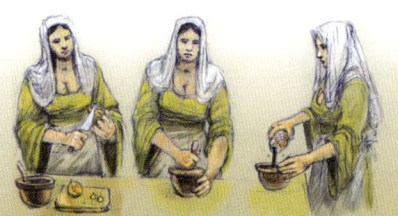

Revision Tip

It is easier to learn information when you reduce it into fewer key points.

Summarise the role of each person who cared for the sick in medieval England on these pages into just three bullet points.

Apply ▶ Recall Challenges

1 Know the key ideas

Match the ideas about the cause of disease and illness on the left with the treatments or preventions on the right.

Ideas about the cause of disease and illness
A punishment from God
Miasma Theory
Astrology
An imbalance of the four humours

Treatment or prevention
Using a star chart to carefully time a treatment
Carrying sweet smelling herbs
Bleeding a patient
Prayer
Removing rotten animals from the streets
Pilgrimage

2 Know the key individuals

Match the questions on the left with the key individuals on the right.

Question
Who treated most people in medieval England when they were sick?
Who treated rich people in medieval England?
Who mixed the herbal remedies used to treat people in medieval England?
Who would often bleed a patient in medieval England?

Key individuals
Physicians
Apothecaries
Barber surgeons
Women

Summarise

Create memory aids to remember key features

A good memory aid:
- answers a key question
- uses minimal words – just key words
- includes a memorable image, diagram or mnemonic.

Here is an example to summarise the information on pages 17–19.

1 Copy the memory aid and add notes to the 4BAG mnemonic so it is ready to be used for revision.
2 Add bullet points to summarise the role of apothecaries, barber surgeons and hospitals in care of the sick.

Key question 1: What did people in the Middle Ages believe caused illness?

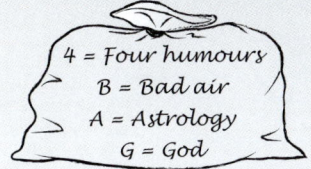

4 = Four humours
B = Bad air
A = Astrology
G = God

Key question 2: Who treated and cared for the sick?

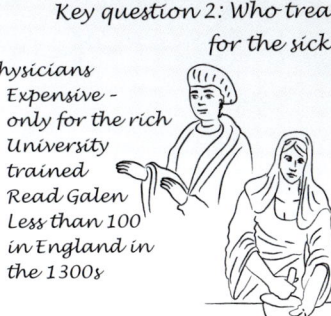

Physicians
- Expensive – only for the rich
- University trained
- Read Galen
- Less than 100 in England in the 1300s

Women
- Treated everyone
- Learned from other women
- If they could read, they used 'herbals' (books which gave them ingredients for remedies)
- Some women trained as barber surgeons

Part 1 Case study: Dealing with the Black Death, 1348–49

> **Research & Record**
>
> **What can the Black Death tell us about medieval medicine?**
> Use pages 24–25 to complete your own copy of a table like this. Record examples of ideas about cause, attempts to prevent its spread and approaches to treatment.
>
> | Ideas about the cause of the Black Death | Attempts to prevent its spread | Approaches to treatment |
> |---|---|---|
> | | | |

Causes: What was the Black Death?

The Black Death was one of the most frightening diseases in history. The map shows how it spread across Europe after arriving from Asia.

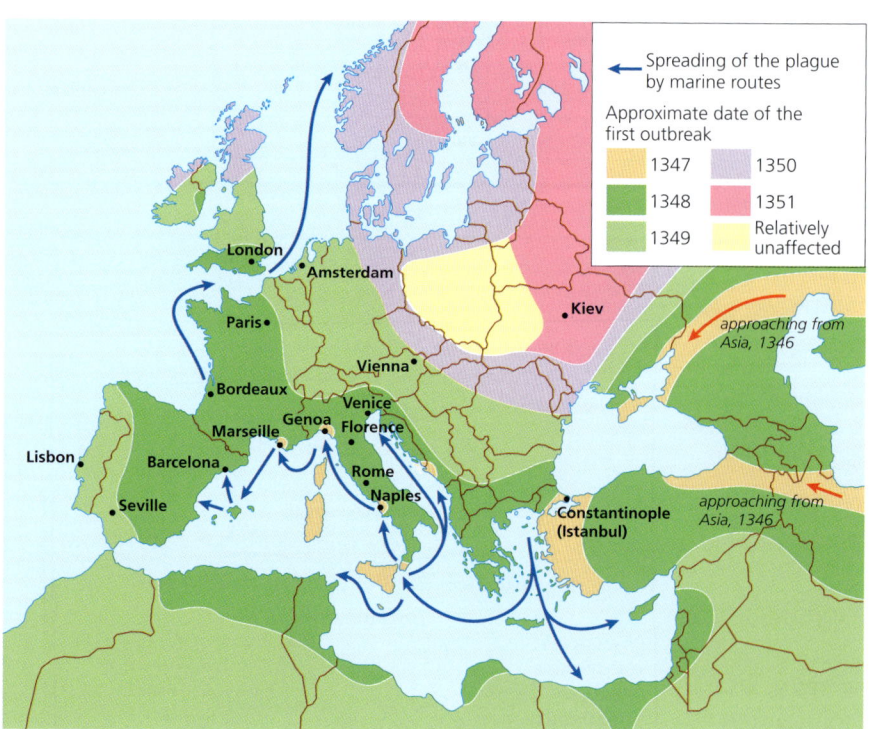

▲ **SOURCE F** The spread of the Black Death by marine routes

It reached England in 1348. Over the next 12 months, historians estimate that the Black Death killed over one-third of the population. Towns and ports were hardest hit. Only remote villages and farms avoided it. The plague affected both rich and poor.

Judging by the way the symptoms were described, historians think the Black Death was a combination of two diseases.

The **main disease** was bubonic plague, carried by rats and spread by fleas. Victims felt cold and tired, then got painful swellings called **buboes**, as big as eggs, on their neck and in their groin or armpits. These were quickly followed by high fever, severe headache, then usually death after three days.

The **epidemic** was probably made worse by pneumonic plague. This was spread by people coughing over others. The disease attacked the lungs. Victims coughed up blood. They died more quickly from this plague than from bubonic plague – in a day or two at most.

Explanations: What did people at the time believe caused it?

God's punishment – the plague was part of God's plan to make people less sinful.

Miasma – bad, stinking air (called miasma) coming from rubbish in the streets spread disease.

Astrology – people became ill because a planet had moved into a new constellation of stars.

The Theory of the Four Humours – people died because they were 'stuffed with evil humours'.

Prevention: How did people try to prevent it from spreading?

There were many different methods. Here is a selection:

- People stopped strangers entering their villages in case they carried the plague.
- New quarantine laws were introduced by the government. People new to an area had to stay away from others for 40 days. However, this law was difficult to enforce.
- Bishops ordered daily services and processions to pray for forgiveness and ask for God's help.
- King Edward III wrote to the Lord Mayor, ordering him to clean the streets. He said that the rubbish was creating 'bad odours' that led to the disease spreading.
- Butchers were punished for leaving the remains of slaughtered animals in the streets.
- People lit huge candles in church as offerings to God.
- People fasted (stopped eating) to show they were sorry for their sins.
- Doors and windows were shut and sealed.
- People went on pilgrimages to pray for God's forgiveness at the tombs of saints.
- People carried sweet-smelling herbs or lit fires to overpower the bad air.
- People kept the air moving by ringing bells or keeping birds to fly around the house.
- Some people punished themselves in public and begged God for forgiveness, as you can see in Source G below.

Treatments: How did people treat its victims?

Historians know very little about the treatments used because, when someone suffered with the plague, they often died very quickly. It is likely there was no time to record the treatments used. However, we do know that the following treatments were used:

- People put charms around the necks of victims.
- Prayers were said for the sick.
- Buboes were cut open to let the pus out.
- It is likely that bleeding would have been used to balance the four humours.
- Herbal remedies were used to cleanse the body, including strong smelling herbs such as aloe and myrrh.

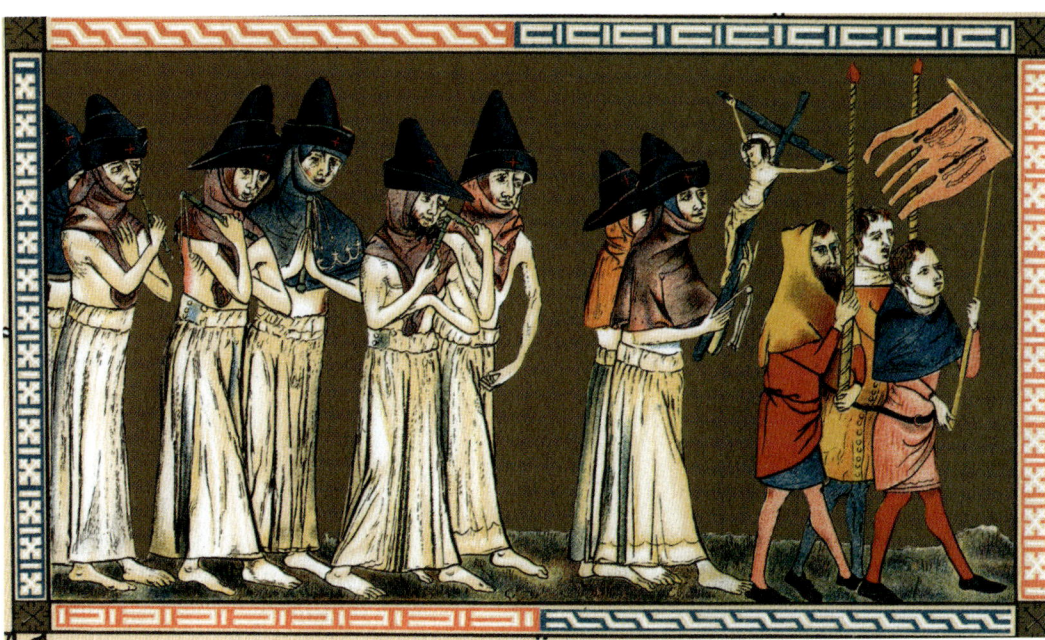

◀ **SOURCE G** This picture shows the Flagellants who arrived in London from Holland. According to the chronicler Robert of Avebury, they walked barefoot through the city twice a day, wearing only a linen cloth. They whipped themselves to show God they had repented their sins and asked God to be merciful

Part 1 Medieval medicine period review

Review 1

Themes

1. The period summary chart below summarises the medieval period. Study it carefully, then create a blank copy (with only the themes listed on the left-hand side) and try to reproduce all the information **from memory alone**. Use a whole page of A4 paper with four rows – one per theme. This is a challenge but worth the effort because it will reveal what you are able to remember easily and what you are finding harder to recall.

2. Once you have done the best you can, review your attempt against our period summary chart. Fill in any gaps using a **different coloured pen**. This will remind you what you are struggling to remember.

Period summary	
Theme	c1250–c1500: Medicine in medieval England
Ideas about the cause of disease and illness	God – a punishment for sins Astrology – movement of the planets Four humours – blood, black bile, yellow bile and phlegm unbalanced Bad air (miasma)
Approaches to prevention	Life free from sin, prayer, confession Keep the air clean and free from miasma by carrying sweet-smelling herbs and removing waste from the streets Exercise, diet and bathing
Approaches to treatment	Prayers, fasting and pilgrimage King's touch Herbal remedies Bloodletting and purging to restore the balance of the humours (Galen's Theory of Opposites) Rest, exercise and diet
Care of the sick	Physicians cared for the rich Apothecaries mixed herbal remedies Barber surgeons performed basic surgery Most people were cared for by women in their family and/or community Hospitals provided care for the elderly and the number increased

Review 2

Importance of the Church

You might need to explain the role played by factors in the development of medicine. Factors can help medicine progress, but they can also lead to continuity.

Look at the example paragraph on the right. It explains how the Church ensured **continuity** in medicine. Note how the highlighted connective 'this meant that' helps to develop the answer – proving that this factor played an important role.

1. Complete this first paragraph, making sure you explain how religious beliefs also discouraged people in medieval England from challenging Galen and developing new ideas.

2. Then, write a second paragraph in which you explain another way in which the Church ensured continuity in medieval medicine. For example, you could explore how Christianity encouraged the establishment of hospitals.

There was continuity in medieval medicine because of the importance of religious beliefs. Throughout the period, people believed that disease and illness were sent by God. During the Black Death, many people believed that it was sent as a punishment from God for their sins. Religious beliefs dominated medicine between c1250 and c1500. This meant that people at the time were discouraged from challenging the ideas of Galen. This was because ....

Summarise

1. On page 23 we used a memory aid similar to the one below to help remember four things that medieval people believed caused disease. Can you remember all four, just by looking at the image?

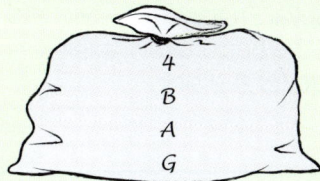

2. Look at the pictures below. What four approaches to prevention and treatment do they show from medieval England?

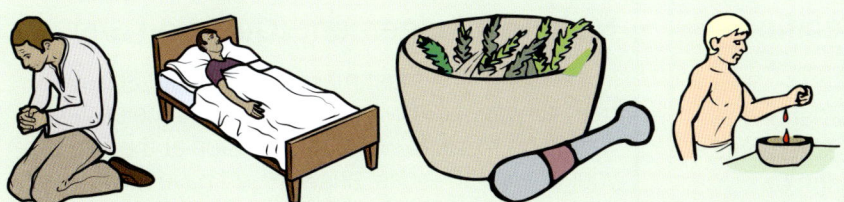

3. Draw and label your own pictures to summarise additional approaches to prevention and treatment.

Medieval medicine exam practice

Revision Tip

Regularly revisit content to make sure it sticks

You have just completed the first part of the course and it may be tempting to move quickly on to Part 2. However, it is important to build in regular revision activities as you progress through your GCSE course.

How do you stop yourself forgetting? The key is to regularly revisit information you have covered. The Recall Challenges below revisit material from this part of the course.

Apply ▶ Recall Challenges

1 Know the key individuals/developments in medicine

a Describe the ideas of Galen.
b Why did Galen's ideas influence medieval medicine?
c Describe hospitals in medieval England.
d What approaches to prevention and treatment did people take during the Black Death?

2 Know the key words

Make an A4 copy of this bingo card. You will need plenty of space to write in each box.

a For each key word/idea, write a definition from memory. Then check your definition against the information in this chapter and in the glossary on pages 133–134.

Key word bingo		
Punishment from God	Theory of the Four Humours	Miasma Theory
Prayer	Bloodletting	Herbal remedies
Physician	Barber surgeon	Apothecary

b For each word on the top row, explain how it was linked to ideas about the cause of disease and illness.
c For each word on the middle row, explain how it was linked to approaches to prevention and treatment in medieval England.
d For each word on the bottom row, explain how the individual cared for the sick.

Exam Tip

Support your answer with specific knowledge

In the exam, you can improve your explanations by including relevant facts to support your arguments. For example, when answering the question on page 29:

- Do not simply describe the Theory of the Four Humours – explain how it influenced approaches to the treatment of disease and illness when people used bloodletting to balance the humours.
- Explain how the Theory of Miasma influenced approaches to preventing the spread of the Black Death in 1348.

Exam Tip

Making a judgement (Question 5/6)

In the exam, you must make a judgement about how far you agree with the statement. The easiest way to do this is to write a conclusion at the end of your answer. The best answers will have their overall judgement running throughout the answer. For example, when answering the question on page 29:

- Decide whether you agree or disagree that medieval medicine was entirely influenced by the ideas of Hippocrates and Galen and begin your paragraph with 'In conclusion, the statement can be disagreed with …'
- Go on to explain why you have reached this judgement by saying that there were other ideas, such as religion and the Theory of Miasma, that also influenced medieval medicine.

Exam Tip

Making a judgement (Question 5/6)

Your exam will include a question that asks you to make a judgement about how far you agree with a statement about causation, consequence, change, continuity or significance.

When you are answering these questions, you should use the **3DS** : **Decode**, **Decide** and **Develop**.

Decode the question (work out the focus of the question).
- Staying focused on the question is crucial. Including information that is not relevant or writing about the wrong topic wastes time and gains no marks.

What are the command words?
The question asks, 'how far do you agree?'. You need to try to agree and disagree with the statement before reaching a judgement.

What is the content focus?
Focus on the ideas of Galen. Weigh these against the other ideas that influenced medicine in medieval England. You need to include at least three aspects of knowledge throughout your answer.

> 'Medieval medicine was entirely influenced by the ideas of **Galen**.'
> **How far do you agree?** Explain your answer.
> You may use the following in your answer:
> - Theory of the Four Humours
> - Religious ideas
>
> You **must** also use information of your own.
>
> **(16 marks)**

What is the conceptual focus?
The historical concept is significance. Describing the ideas of Galen is not enough to get the higher-level marks. Focus on explaining why you agree and disagree that their ideas influenced medicine in medieval England and then support with examples from your knowledge.

How many marks are available?
'16 marks' indicates you should spend about 24 minutes on the question. You should try to write at least three paragraphs: at least one paragraph that agrees with the statement, at least one that disagrees and a conclusion.

There are also 4 marks for SPAG. This means your spelling, punctuation and grammar. Check that you have used capital letters, commas, full stops and paragraphs correctly.

Decide how to organise your answer into paragraphs.
You do not have the time to tell the story of medieval medicine. The focus is on the influence of the ideas of Galen in this period. Decide the main arguments you want to explain and then organise these reasons into three paragraphs. One possible approach is:
- Paragraph 1: Agree with the statement – explain how the ideas of Galen, in particular the Theory of the Four Humours, influenced medieval medicine.
- Paragraph 2: Disagree with the statement – explain that there were other ideas that influenced medieval medicine, such as Miasma Theory.
- Paragraph 3: Disagree with the statement again – explain how religious ideas also influenced medieval medicine, such as the idea that illness was believed to be sent by God as a punishment for sin.
- Paragraph 4: End with a conclusion - decide if you agree or disagree with the statement overall and explain why.

Develop your answer in relation to the question.
- Make sure you explain and support the points you make. Do not simply state that the ideas of Galen influenced medieval medicine – explain how and give specific examples.
- Do not simply state that other ideas influenced medieval medicine. Explain these ideas and explain that they were not influenced by Galen.

Part 2 Ideas about the cause of disease and illness c1500–c1700

Connect & Engage – Andreas Vesalius

Andreas Vesalius was born in Belgium in 1514. He studied medicine in Italy, becoming Professor of Surgery at Padua University at the age of just 22. Vesalius lived during a period known as the Renaissance, a time when old ideas were being questioned. He respected Galen's work but believed it was vital to ask questions and challenge traditional ideas by carrying out dissections. He had to be inventive and determined. Once, he stole the body of a criminal from the gallows to dissect. After that, a local judge agreed to give him the bodies of executed criminals so that he could study the structure of the body more closely.

Vesalius published his work in *De Humani Corporis Fabrica (On the Fabric of the Human Body)* in 1543. He proved that Galen had made some mistakes:

- The human jaw bone is made from one bone, not two as Galen had said.
- The breastbone has three parts, not seven as Galen had said.
- Blood does not flow into the heart through invisible holes in the **septum** – such holes do not exist.

Vesalius' book was full of illustrations showing the body in far more detail and more accurately than had ever been done before. The invention of the printing press meant the book was widely available to doctors all over Europe. By the 1560s, it was being used in England to train doctors and correct mistakes in older medical books.

His book also encouraged doctors to carry out their own dissections. The first recorded public dissection in England was carried out in 1565 by an anatomist in Cambridge. However, many doctors stuck to traditional ideas, not daring to think for themselves, still saying it was wrong to challenge Galen. Vesalius faced lots of criticism and was forced to leave Padua University.

Connect & Engage

How did a Belgian studying in Italy influence medicine in England?

Complete your own table like the one below to record Vesalius' impact.

Area of medicine	Impact? Yes/No	Explanation (include whether his work had impact in the short term or the long term)
Ideas about the cause of disease and illness		
Approaches to prevention		
Approaches to treatment		
Knowledge of the body		
Medical training		

The influence of Vesalius in England

Before Vesalius – the story so far

In the Middle Ages:
- Medical training was based on books written by Galen.
- The study of anatomy had almost disappeared; doctors were taught that Galen had given a fully correct description of anatomy so there was no point trying to find things out for themselves.
- Dissection was carried out to show that Galen was right, not to challenge him.

Vesalius' key ideas/key findings

- **Knowledge**: Correcting mistakes made by Galen.
- **Attitudes**: The importance of dissection and asking questions.

Short-term impact (the next 30 years)

- Vesalius' book quickly improved knowledge about anatomy around Europe.
- It helped change attitudes. Some doctors realised there was more to be learned.
- It helped change training. Some doctors carried out human (not animal) dissection to learn more.
- It triggered other research into anatomy. Using the approach outlined by Vesalius, one of his students (Falloppio) published a book showing the structure of the human skull and ear.

But…

LIMITATIONS

- No one was healthier as a result of Vesalius' work.
- He did not affect understanding of disease or treatments. For most of the period c1500–c1700, doctors still based their treatments on Galen and other ancient writers.
- Even in 1668, Samuel Pepys noted in his diary that the leading expert on eye problems in London had only ever seen animals' eyes dissected, never a human eye.

Long-term impact (the next 300 years)

- Gradually, other doctors followed Vesalius' example and started to challenge traditional ideas in other areas of medicine. In the seventeenth century, William Harvey proved – through dissection and experiments – how the heart circulates blood around the body.
- Vesalius' insistence on enquiry was a turning point. By the late 1600s, most students were encouraged to find things out themselves and gain hands-on experience of dissections.

Revision Tip

A good memory aid summarises the key points in as few words as possible and has a mnemonic or a drawing to help trigger memory.

A = Anatomy (the main area of medicine that Vesalius worked in)
B = Book (*On the Fabric of the Human Body* spread this knowledge)
C = Challenged (traditional ideas – particularly Galen)
D = Dissection (showed the importance of dissecting human bodies)
E = Education (doctors should learn by finding out things for themselves – rather than just by reading books)

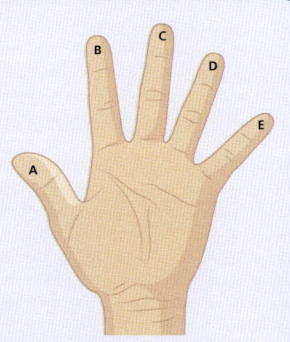

▲ The ABCDE of Vesalius

Continuity and change in explanations of the cause of disease

Research & Record

How much did ideas about the cause of disease and illness change in the years c1500 to c1700?

1. As you read through pages 32–33, use a table like this to record the ideas that existed about the cause of disease and illness.
2. Then evaluate how much change this period saw in ideas about the cause of disease and illness. Choose the appropriate phrase from the scale below and explain why you have come to this conclusion.

Evidence of continuity in ideas about the cause of disease and illness	Evidence of change in ideas about the cause of disease and illness

A total change in … — Significant change — Some changes but mainly continuity — Considerable continuity — No change in …

3. Choose the strongest piece of evidence to support your overall conclusion.

What was the Renaissance?

The word 'Renaissance' is French and means re-birth. The Medical Renaissance was a period when old ideas were being questioned and new ideas were beginning to influence medicine. The classical ideas of people such as Galen began to be challenged. It was the beginning of new scientific ideas.

The changes England experienced during the Renaissance had an impact on the understanding of the cause of illness, as well as prevention and treatment. New inventions, such as the microscope, helped make new discoveries. Inventions such as the printing press helped to share these new ideas quickly and further.

Revision Tip

The factors that held back or led to change should be considered at all stages of your revision. You could make notes under relevant factors for each period. For the Medical Renaissance, write notes under the following headings, giving details of each of these during this period and how they either prevented or brought about change in these years.

- Individuals
- The Church
- Science and technology
- Attitudes in society

Old ideas continue

Old ideas about the cause of disease and illness continued during the Medical Renaissance in England. These ideas included that disease and illness occurred because of an imbalance of the four humours and were spread by miasma (bad smells). The idea that disease was spread by miasma was believed more widely during an epidemic, such as the Great Plague in 1665.

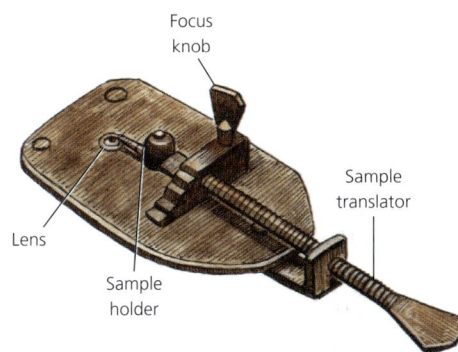

▲ SOURCE A The early Leeuwenhoek microscope

New discoveries

Some people came up with new scientific discoveries. From 1683, more powerful microscopes, developed by Antoni van Leeuwenhoek, were being used. These enabled the first recorded observation of bacteria. Tiny animalcules (a word used to describe what were thought to be tiny animals before bacteria was discovered) were seen in plaque scraped from between the teeth, but the images were not very clear. More importantly, nobody made the connection between **microbes** and disease so the discovery was an important step, but it had limited impact on the understanding of the cause of disease or its treatment.

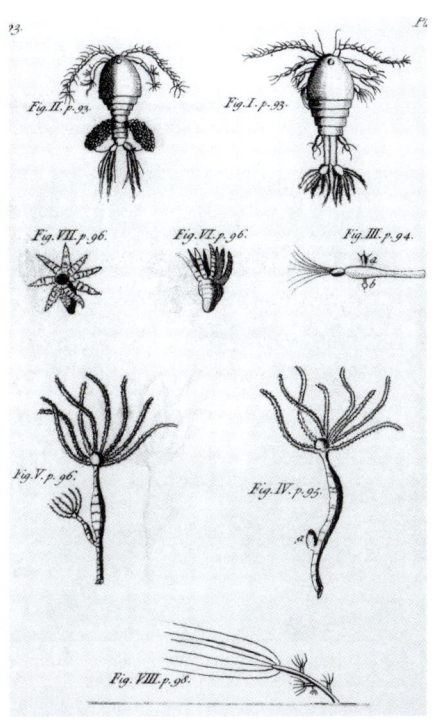

▲ SOURCE B Antoni van Leeuwenhoek's drawing of what he called 'little animals' under the microscope, published in 1677. This was the first recorded sighting of microorganisms

Religion

During this period, most people began to change their views and began to believe that disease and illness were not sent as a punishment by God. However, the old beliefs could be reawakened by a major disaster. For example, during the Great Plague of 1665, there were many pamphlets and preachers claiming that the plague was sent by God.

Apply ▶ Exam Practice

Question 5/6 style

Use the information on this page alongside the information on pages 16, 25 and 46 to answer the question below. Remind yourself of how to answer this type of exam question using the advice on page 29.

'There was little progress in understanding the cause of disease in the years c1250 to c1700.' How far do you agree? Explain your answer. (16 marks)

You may use the following in your answer:
- Miasma Theory
- The Great Plague in London, 1665

You **must** also use information of your own.

Exam Tip

Dates

Check the dates in the question carefully to make sure that you are writing about the correct chronological period in the history of medicine in Britain. This question refers to c1250 to c1700 so you need to use your knowledge of medieval medicine and the Medical Renaissance.

Improvements in a scientific approach and the transmission of ideas

Research & Record

Why was there progress in the understanding of the cause of disease and illness during the Medical Renaissance?

Use a table like this to explain why there were developments in the understanding of the cause of disease and illness during the Medical Renaissance.

You will need to add to your table after reading pages 42–43, so leave lots of space.

Complete the explanations (column 2) for all of the reasons before you complete the evaluations (column 3).

Reason	Explanation How did it lead to progress in understanding of the cause of disease and illness?	Evaluation How important was it for understanding the cause of disease and illness?
The impact of individuals		
Developments in technology		
Developments in scientific understanding		

The work of Thomas Sydenham

Thomas Sydenham was a doctor who made progress in the diagnosis of disease and illness. He believed in careful observation of the patient and of the illness. As a result, he gained the name the 'English Hippocrates'. The work of Thomas Sydenham was important in moving medicine away from the ideas of Galen and Hippocrates, and into the new scientific era.

Sydenham was educated at Oxford and Cambridge universities before becoming a physician in London. As a physician, he told young doctors, 'You must go to the bedside. It is there alone that you can learn about disease.' He believed that a doctor should take a more scientific approach, which included taking a full history of the patient's health and symptoms. He also believed that before diagnosing the patient's illness, the doctor should examine them carefully, for example by listening to their pulse. Thomas Sydenham believed that each disease was different and should be identified carefully so that the correct treatment could be prescribed. He was therefore rejecting the idea that all disease could be understood with a single theory like the Theory of the Four Humours.

Sydenham made detailed descriptions of many illnesses. His first description was of scarlet fever. This led Sydenham to contribute to the long-term progress of medicine in this period. Sydenham discovered that measles and scarlet fever were different diseases, but he was unable to discover the different **microorganisms** that caused the diseases. He published his findings in many books which led to his ideas being shared more widely. His most famous book was probably *Observationes Medicae* (*Observations of Medicine*), published in 1676.

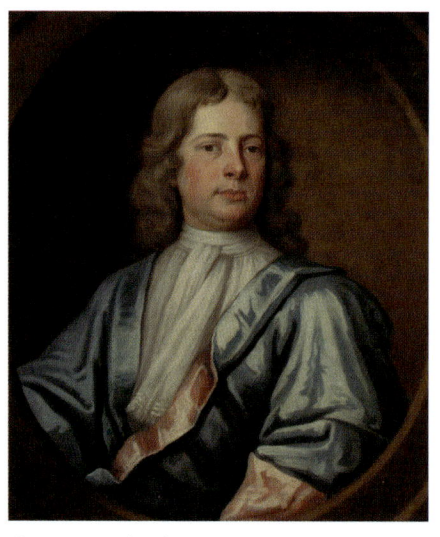

▲ A portrait of Thomas Sydenham (1624–89)

The influence of the printing press

One piece of technology had a massive impact on medicine, even though it had nothing to do with doctors or disease. In the 1450s, a German man, Johannes Gutenberg, built the first printing press. A printing press was a machine that would print text and pictures. This meant that books no longer had to be written by hand. Many copies of the same text could be printed and ideas shared more widely. By 1500, there were printing presses across Europe.

The availability of new information and ideas had a huge impact on the understanding and treatment of disease. The printing press enabled new medical ideas to be transmitted accurately and quickly. Scientists were able to publish and share their discoveries.

At the same time, the Church had much less control over what information was shared and could not prevent ideas they disapproved of from being published. Physicians were now able to publish ideas that challenged the work of Galen.

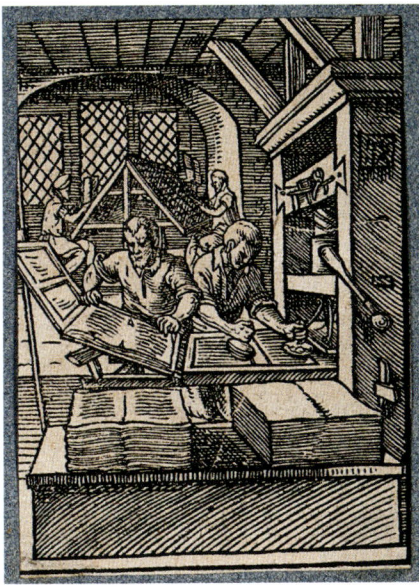

▲ **SOURCE C** A woodcut showing the printing press in 1568

The work of The Royal Society

From 1645, meetings took place in London of a group of people who wanted to discuss new ideas in science. Discussions also took place about medicine. They had their own laboratory where they carried out experiments, and they published books to spread their ideas. From 1662, this group became known as The Royal Society because King Charles II attended their talks. His support for their ideas helped to influence others to provide financial and political support for their schemes. People donated to The Royal Society so that their work could continue. Probably the biggest impact of The Royal Society was through its publications. Each year they published their *Philosophical Transactions*, which recorded the scientific developments its members had been involved in or had heard about.

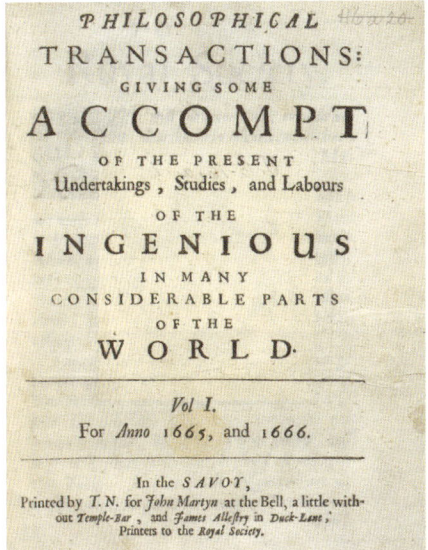

▲ **SOURCE D** The cover page of The Royal Society's *Transactions* 1665–66

Exam Tip

Support your answer with specific knowledge

In the exam, you can improve your explanations by including relevant facts to support your arguments. For example, instead of writing 'Thomas Sydenham was important', you could write:

Thomas Sydenham was important in encouraging other doctors to question and challenge traditional ideas about the cause of disease and illness. His approach to observing the patient and the illness led to him discovering that measles and scarlet fever were different diseases.

Part 2 Approaches to prevention and treatment c1500–c1700

Continuity and change in approaches to prevention and treatment

Research & Record

How far did approaches to prevention and treatment change in the years c1500 to c1700?

Read pages 36–38 and gather evidence to support the arguments in the table below. You will be able to use these notes to answer the exam questions on page 39.

Argument	Support
Approaches to prevention and treatment changed in the years c1500 to c1700.	Scientists began to look for chemical cures and experimented with metal, such as mercury.
Approaches to prevention and treatment remained unchanged in the years c1500 to c1700.	Treatments based on the Theory of the Four Humours continued, such as bloodletting.

Miasma Theory

People continued to base their efforts to prevent disease and illness on their beliefs in theories such as the Miasma Theory. Cleanliness was seen as a way to avoid miasma (bad air). Fines were issued to homeowners who did not keep the street outside of their house clean.

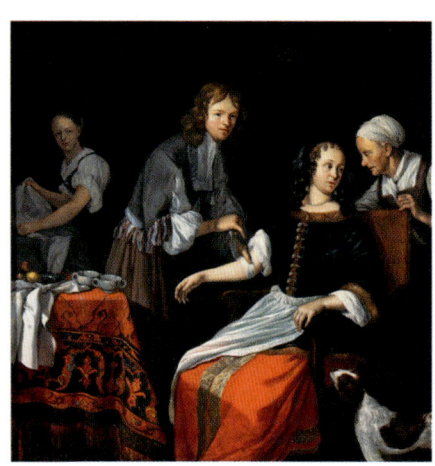

▲ **SOURCE E** This painting by a Dutch artist shows a physician binding up a woman's arm after bloodletting. It was painted in 1666. You can see the bleeding cup on the table

Bloodletting and purging

Treatments aimed at balancing the four humours continued, such as bloodletting and purging. These were meant to correct the balance in the body, though they must have weakened the patient. When King Charles II was sick in 1685, this was the main treatment used on him. This tells us that it was still prioritised as a treatment for illness during this period.

Herbal remedies

Herbal remedies continued to be used to treat disease and illness. Home remedies were handed down through generations from mother to daughter. Local plants and products from animals were used for medicines and ointments to treat injuries and illnesses.

The printing revolution meant that more people learned to read and could buy 'herbals' (books with advice on herbal remedies). One of the most popular books was *Complete Herbal* by Nicholas Culpepper, which described the properties of herbs that could be used at home and which parts of the body or which ailments they were good for. Culpepper also linked each herb to one of the signs of the zodiac or one of the planets.

New treatments from abroad

As new countries were discovered by the West during this period, new herbs were brought back to England. For example:

- Rhubarb from Asia was widely used to purge the bowels.
- The bark of the cinchona tree from South America was used to treat fevers. In Europe, it became known as **quinine** and helped many who suffered from malaria.
- Less helpfully, opium from Turkey was used as an anaesthetic. It worked, but it was highly addictive and easy to overdose.
- Tobacco was greeted as a **'cure-all'** when it arrived from America, being recommended for toothache, poisoned wounds, joint pains and as protection from plague. One schoolboy commented that during the Plague of 1665, he was beaten for 'not smoking often enough'.

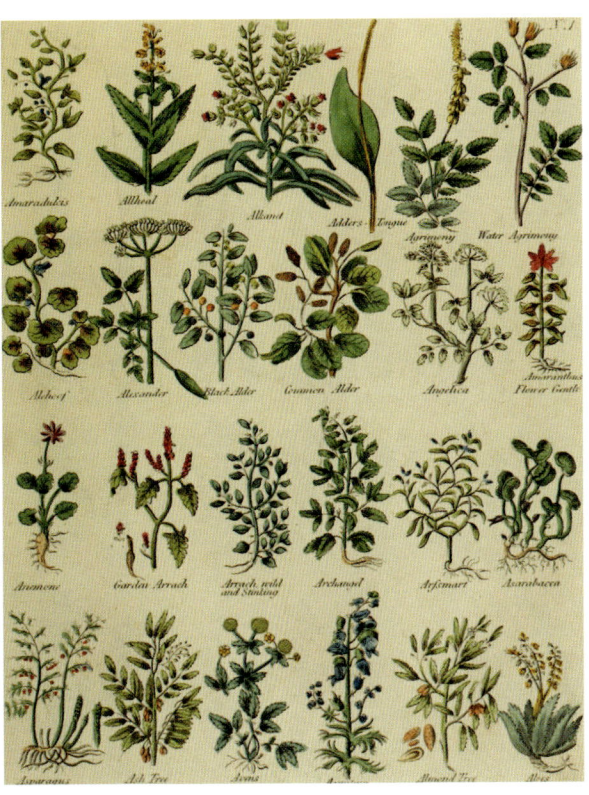

▲ **SOURCE F** An image from Nicholas Culpepper's *Complete Herbal* showing the homegrown herbal remedies that were recommended

Apply ▶ Recall Challenges

Revisiting Part 1

Remember it is important to regularly revisit what you have learnt. Look back at the Recall Challenges at the end of Part 1 (see page 28). Try to complete these again from memory before checking your answers.

Testing yourself on Part 2

Know the key words

Make an A4 copy of this bingo card. You will need plenty of space to write in each box.

Key word bingo		
Theory of the Four Humours	Microscope	Punishment from God
Miasma Theory	Animalcules	Scarlet fever
The Royal Society	Herbal remedies	Bloodletting

a For each key word, write a definition from memory. Then check your definition against the information in this chapter and the glossary on pages 133–134.

b Which key words can you use to explain the continuity in medical ideas about the cause of disease and illness from medieval to Renaissance England?

c Which key words can you use to explain the change in medical ideas about the cause of disease and illness from medieval to Renaissance England?

d Which key words can you use to explain the continuity in approaches to prevention and treatment from medieval to Renaissance England?

e Which key words can you use to explain the change in approaches to prevention and treatment from medieval to Renaissance England?

Chemical cures

The growth in science during the Renaissance led people to look for chemical cures. Medical professionals began to experiment with metals, such as mercury, as cures. These people were called alchemists.

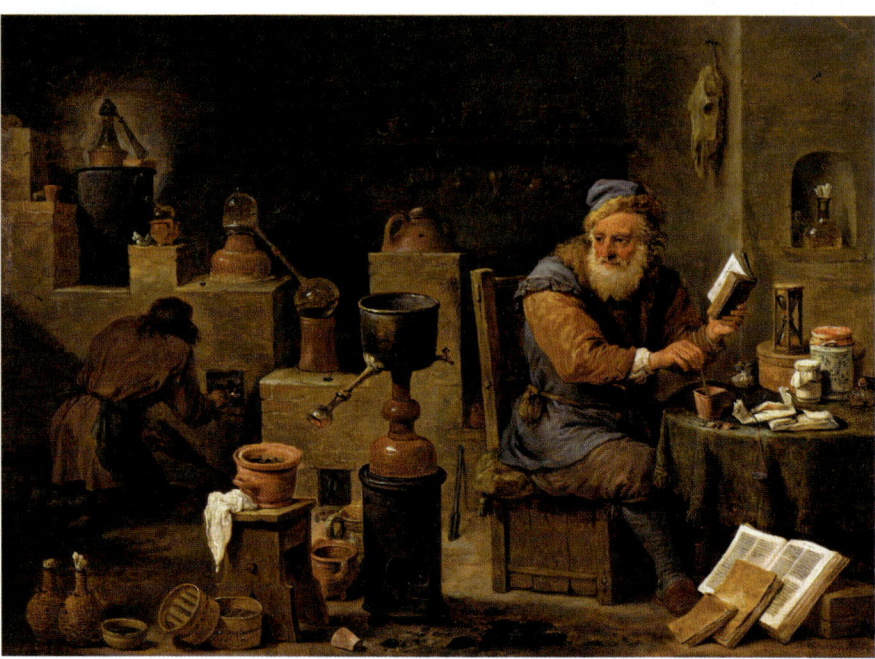

▲ **SOURCE G** *The Alchemist,* by David Teniers the Younger, seventeenth century

Transference

A popular idea that developed during the Renaissance was transference. It was believed that an illness or disease could be transferred from the victim to something else. People believed that if you rubbed an object on the symptom of the illness, such as a boil, the illness would transfer to the object.

Treatments based on superstition

It was still believed that the King could cure scrofula, a skin disease, by touching a victim. Between 1660 and 1682, over 92,000 people visited the King's court in the hope of being cured of the 'King's Evil'.

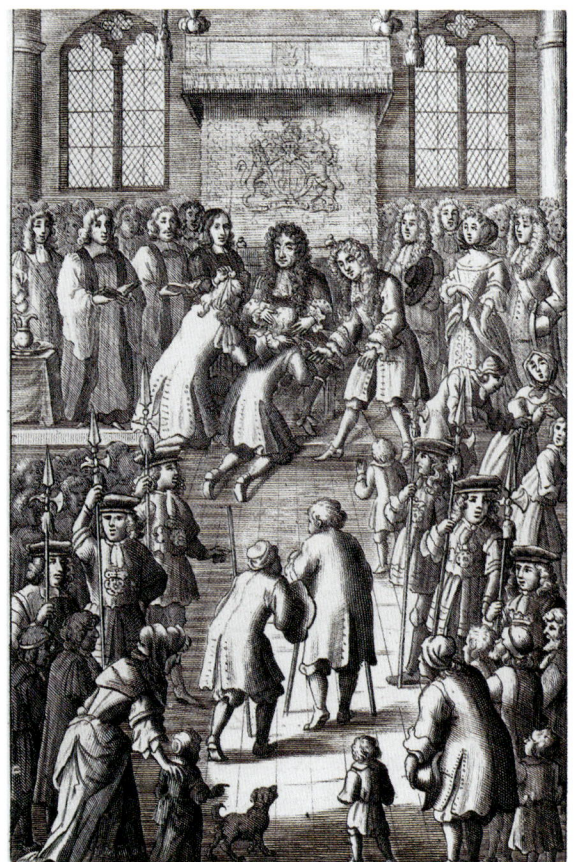

◀ **SOURCE H** This engraving shows people being touched by Charles II

Apply ▶ Exam Practice

Question 3 style

Use the Exam Tip to help you answer these questions:
- Explain **one** way in which the approaches to the treatment of disease and illness in the period c1250 to c1500 were similar to the approaches to the treatment of disease and illness in the period c1500 to c1700.
- Explain **one** way in which the attempts to prevent disease and illness in the period c1250 to c1500 were similar to the attempts to prevent disease and illness in the period c1500 to c1700.

Exam Tip

Comparing time periods (Question 3)

Use the steps below to help you answer the questions in the Exam Practice box.

Step 1: Identify the **content focus** of the question. Both questions compare **one feature** (**the treatment of disease and illness** or **the prevention of disease and illness**) in two different time periods.

Step 2: Identify the **conceptual focus** of the question. Focus on **similarity**. Do not go into differences.

Step 3: **Write**. You will have about six minutes for this type of 4-mark question. Aim for four or five sentences. Identify the similarity and develop this with explanation. Include an example from both periods.

See the possible answer to the first question. Choose some different examples in your answer to this question.

Possible answer

During the period c1250 to c1500 people would treat disease and illness with herbal remedies. Herbal remedies used in this period included aloe vera, camomile, rose, oils and mint. Herbal remedies continued to be used in the period c1500 to c1700. By this time new countries had been discovered by the West and new herbs were brought back to England, including the bark of the cinchona tree from South America, which was used to treat fevers.

- 'A similar approach to the treatment of disease in both time periods has been identified – herbal remedies'.
- 'This is supported with an example from both time periods'

Revision Tip

As you learn about medicine in Britain from c1250 to the present day it is important to look for examples of change and continuity in:
- the ideas about the cause of disease and illness
- approaches to prevention and treatment of disease and illness.

For the Medical Renaissance, write notes under the these headings, giving examples of change and continuity for the period. You could organise this information in tables – one for each heading. You can challenge yourself by explaining why there was change and/or continuity.

Continuity and change in care of the sick

> ### Research & Record
>
> **How much continuity was there in the care given by the community and in hospitals?**
> Complete a table like this using information on pages 40–41.
>
> | Key questions | Medieval England | Renaissance England | Evaluation/extent of change |
> |---|---|---|---|
> | Who cared for the sick? | | | |
> | Where were the sick cared for? | | | |

Treatment and care in the community

The same people offered medical treatment in England during the Renaissance: physicians, apothecaries and barber surgeons.

Most sick people continued to be cared for at home. This meant that women continued to play a significant role, as midwives, mixing herbal remedies and caring for the sick. Those who could afford to paid for a doctor or nurse to care for them at home.

Treatment and care in hospitals

There were fewer hospitals available in England after the dissolution of the monasteries. In 1534, Henry VIII made himself Head of the Church in England rather than the Pope. One measure he brought in was the dissolution (closing down) of the monasteries because he disapproved of them and wanted their wealth. This had a damaging effect on poor people and the sick as many hospitals were lost. Some smaller hospitals did open, usually paid for by charities, but there were not as many as before the dissolution.

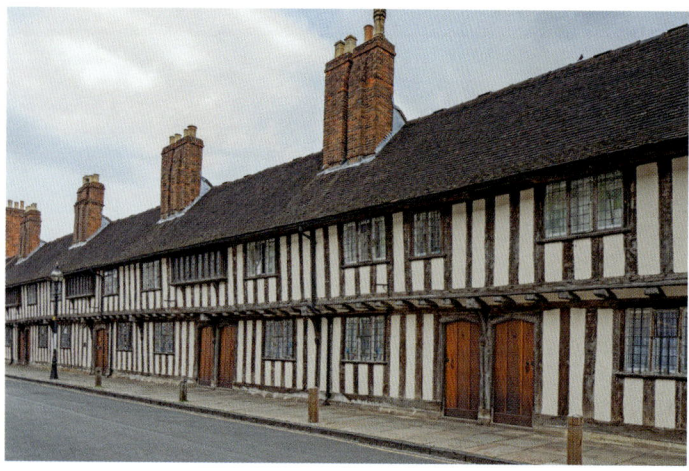

▲ **SOURCE I** Almshouses in Stratford upon Avon, built in the sixteenth century

Some hospitals were taken over by town councils, especially the **almshouses** that looked after the elderly poor. In London, the city council and charity helped to keep St Bartholomew's Hospital open. By the 1660s, it had 12 wards and up to 300 patients, looked after by three physicians.

Monks and nuns continued to care for those in hospitals linked to the Church. However, evidence suggests that there was a change in the care given in hospitals during the Medical Renaissance. People went to hospitals with wounds and diseases, such as fevers and skin conditions. At some hospitals, physicians came to visit patients and in a few, the physicians worked there all the time.

Pest houses

One change that did take place in this period was the introduction of pest houses. These were buildings where people suffering from one particular disease, such as **smallpox**, were looked after. They emerged as people realised that disease could be passed from one person to another. The intention was to keep people with these diseases away from the rest of the community. Other names used for these buildings were 'plague houses' and 'pox houses'.

Improvements in medical training

For most of the period between c1500 and c1700, physicians still learned about medicine from the work and books of Galen. However, in the late 1600s this began to change.

- In some hospitals, such as in Edinburgh, training took place on the wards.
- Medical training led to students being taught more about correct anatomy due to the work of Vesalius and Harvey (see pages 30–31 and 42–43).
- The scientific approach of asking questions and observation was emphasised.
- More dissections took place as they were no longer banned by the Church.
- New equipment was developed and became available, such as microscopes and thermometers.

Apply ▶ Exam Practice

Question 3 style

1 Explain **one** way in which the care of the sick in the years c1250 to c1500 was similar to the care of the sick in the years c1500 to c1700. (4 marks)
2 Explain **one** way in which the care of the sick in the years c1250 to c1500 was different to the care of the sick in the years c1500 to c1700. (4 marks)

Exam Tip

Comparing time periods (Question 3)

Look again at the advice on how to approach this type of question on page 39.

Remember to focus on explaining a similarity/difference and supporting your explanation with an example from both time periods. Think about:
- who treated the sick
- where the sick were cared for.

Part 2 Case study: William Harvey and the discovery of the circulation of the blood

Research & Record

What contribution did William Harvey make to the Medical Renaissance?

The table below shows the approach to anatomical knowledge before the Medical Renaissance in England. Copy the table and complete the right-hand column with details of William Harvey's discovery and its significance as you read pages 42–43.

Anatomical knowledge before the Medical Renaissance in England	William Harvey's discovery and its significance
Galen developed his ideas by dissecting pigs and apes.	
Galen believed that blood was continually created by the liver to replace the blood burned up in the body.	
Galen believed that the veins carried blood and air around the body.	
Galen believed that blood passed via invisible holes in the septum from one side of the heart to the other.	
Over 300 books of Galen's ideas were published.	
Medical professionals used Galen's books to learn about the anatomy of the human body.	
Galen's ideas were not questioned because they were supported by the Church	

William Harvey was born in 1578. He studied medicine at Cambridge and at Padua in Italy. He returned to London to work as a doctor and became the doctor to King Charles I, which showed how well respected he had become. You had to be a good doctor to be employed by the King!

In 1628 Harvey published his book *An Anatomical Account of the Motion of the Heart and Blood in Animals*. Harvey had discovered how blood circulates around the body and he described this in his book. Harvey proved that the heart acted as a pump and pumped blood around the body.

Previous knowledge

Up until Harvey's discovery, the ideas of Galen were believed. Galen thought that:

- Blood was continually created by the liver to replace the blood burned up in the body.

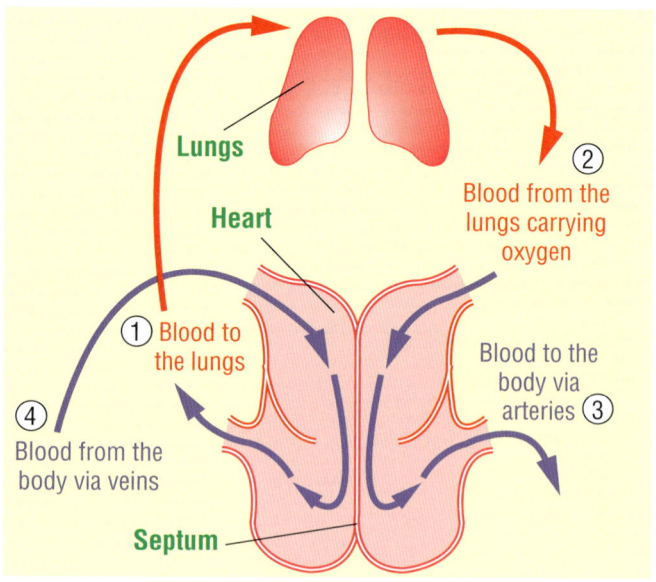

▲ **SOURCE J** A simplified version of the circulation of the blood. Blood leaves the heart (1), then passes through the lungs (2) and back to the heart and then around the body along arteries (3). Then blood comes back to the heart along veins (4) before starting its circulation around the body again

- Veins carried blood and air around the body.
- Blood passed via invisible holes in the septum from one side of the heart to the other.

Proving Galen was wrong

As we know, Vesalius had already started to prove the ideas of Galen were wrong. Harvey continued the work of Vesalius by questioning the ideas of Galen and observing the human body closely.

Harvey carried out a range of scientific experiments to make his discovery:

- He dissected cold-blooded animals, such as frogs, because their heartbeat is slower. This enabled Harvey to see every muscle in the heart move.
- He dissected human bodies to gain a detailed knowledge of the heart.
- Harvey proved that blood flowed in one direction. He was unable to pump liquid past the valves in the veins.
- Harvey proved that the veins carry blood but not air, as Galen had said.
- Harvey calculated the amount of blood inside of a human body to show that the same blood was pumped around the body to the heart.

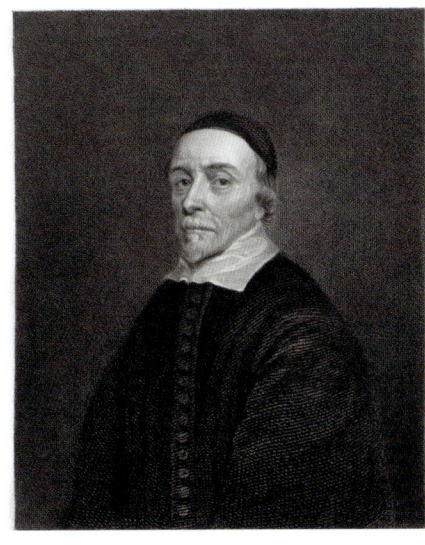

▲ A portrait of William Harvey (1578–1657)

The significance of Harvey's discovery

In many respects, Harvey's discovery was hugely significant:

- Harvey was the first to gain an accurate understanding of the circulation of blood around the body. His work laid the foundations for further study of how the human body worked.
- With the help of The Royal Society, Harvey published his ideas and they were read by other scientists and doctors.
- Harvey's discovery enabled further discoveries in other areas of medicine, for example, surgery.
- Harvey encouraged other scientists and doctors to carry out dissections and look closely at the human body.

However, there were factors which limited the impact of Harvey's discoveries:

- Harvey did not have the technology to discover everything. It was not until microscopes were developed that **capillaries** were discovered. This discovery explained how blood moves from the arteries to the veins.
- Harvey's discovery only had limited impact because it did not improve knowledge of the cause of illness and disease. No preventions or treatments were developed as a result.

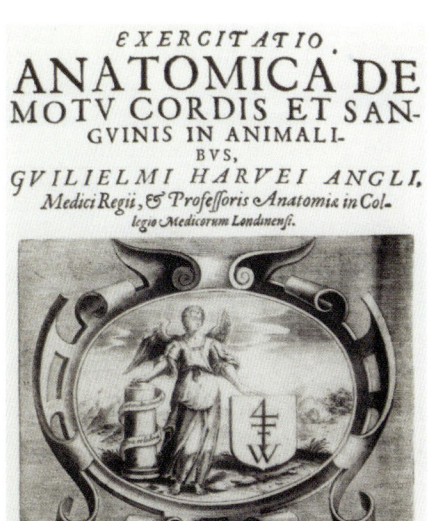

▲ **SOURCE K** The cover page of Harvey's book on the circulation of the blood

Apply ▶ Recall Challenges

1 Know the key individuals
Look at these key individuals:
- Claudius Galen
- Thomas Sydenham
- Andreas Vesalius
- William Harvey

For each one, try to answer these questions from memory:
- In what time period were they important?
- What were their ideas and beliefs about medicine?
- Why were they important? What impact did they have on medicine?

2 Know the key events
Look at these key events:
- Invention of the microscope
- Invention of the printing press
- Creation of The Royal Society
- Dissolution of the monasteries
- Discovery of the circulation of the blood

For each one, try to answer these questions from memory:
- When did the event happen?
- What happened? (Aim to remember at least two factual details.)
- Why did the event happen?
- What were the consequences of the event? What impact did it have on medicine?

3 Know the key words
Make an A4 copy of this bingo card. You will need plenty of space to write in each box.

Key word bingo		
Renaissance	Anatomy	Microscope
Printing press	Transference	Microorganisms
Pest house	Cure-all	Capillaries
New inventions	New ideas about medicine	Care in the community
Change	Supernatural ideas	Dissection

a For each key word on the first three rows, try to write a definition of the word **from memory**, without looking anything up. Then check with the information on this page and in the glossary on pages 133–134.
b For each word on the fourth row, give as many examples as you can.
c For each word on the fifth row, give the opposite.

Apply ▶ Exam Practice

Question 4 style

Use your research from this chapter and the Exam Tip on page 45 to answer the exam question below.

Explain why there were improvements in medical knowledge in the years c1500–c1700. (12 marks)

Exam Tip

Explaining change or continuity (Question 4)

Your exam will include a question that asks you to explain why change took place.

Remember to use the **3Ds**.

Decode the question (work out the focus of the question).

- Including information that is not relevant or writing about the wrong topic wastes time and gains no marks.

What are the command words?
The question starts 'explain why'. You need to explain at least one reason.

What is the content focus?
Focus on the improvements in medical knowledge. You need to include at least three aspects of supporting knowledge throughout your answer.

> **Explain why** there were **improvements in medical knowledge** in the years c1500–c1700. **(12 marks)**

What is the conceptual focus?
The historical concept is causation. Describing medical knowledge is not enough to get the higher-level marks. Focus on explaining why there were improvements in medical knowledge and then support with examples from your knowledge.

How many marks are available?
'12 marks' indicates you should spend about 18 minutes on the question and write no more than three paragraphs (one per aspect of supporting knowledge).

Decide how to organise your answer into paragraphs.

You do not have the time to tell the story of the Medical Renaissance. The focus is on the improvements in medical knowledge. Decide the main reasons you want to explain and then organise these reasons into three paragraphs. One possible approach is:

- Paragraph 1: The importance of the scientific approach – explain how Sydenham questioned and challenged the existing approach to medical diagnosis.
- Paragraph 2: The importance of the scientific approach – explain how Vesalius and Harvey challenged Galen's ideas through careful experimentation and dissection.
- Paragraph 3: The importance of new technology – explain how the printing press enabled new medical ideas to be shared more widely.

Develop your answer by explaining and supporting the points you make.

- Do not simply state that Sydenham questioned the existing approach to medical diagnosis – explain how and give specific examples.
- Do not simply state that Vesalius and Harvey challenged the ideas of Galen. Explain why this was important and how it changed medical training.

Case study: William Harvey and the discovery of the circulation of the blood

45

Part 2 Case Study: Dealing with the Great Plague in London, 1665

Research & Record

How far were responses to the 1665 Plague similar to those to the Black Death?

In the exam, Question 3 tests your ability to compare two events or developments from different time periods. This activity will help you practise comparison.

1. How much can you remember about the Black Death? Try to fill in the second column of a table like this from memory alone.
2. Check what you have written against your research notes and pages 24–25. Fill in any gaps and correct any errors.
3. Use these pages 46–48 to fill in the third column.
4. Reflect on what you have found out:
   - Looking at the two events, what are the similarities in the ideas about cause, and approaches to treatment and prevention?
   - Why were responses to the two events so similar?

	The Black Death, 1348–49	The Great Plague, 1665
Ideas about cause		
Approaches to treatment		
Attempts to prevent its spread		

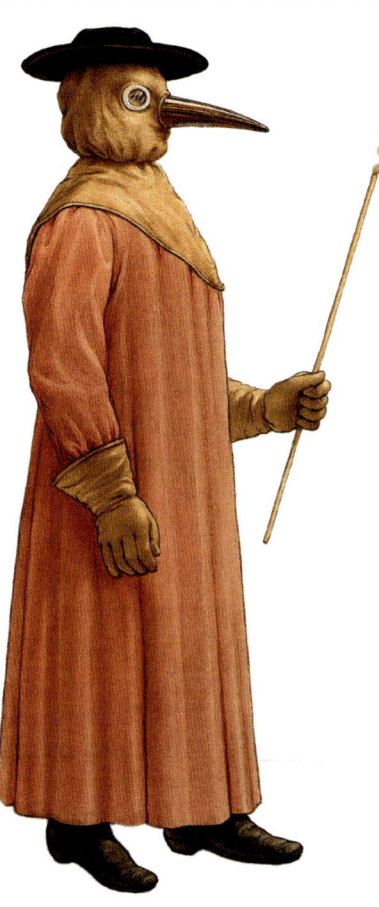

Plague did not disappear after the Black Death of 1348–49. It continued to disrupt England for hundreds of years afterwards. Plague returned to Leicester in the 1550s and 1640s, to London in 1603 and to York in 1604. However, the next time the plague killed thousands of people all over Britain was in 1665. We call this the Great Plague. In London, it killed 75,000 people.

Explanations: What did people think caused the Great Plague?

Many people still believed that God had sent plague to punish them for their sins. The government ordered days of public prayer and fasting so that people could publicly confess their sins and beg God to be merciful.

Others blamed the movements of planets or poisonous air, just as in the Black Death of 1348–49. If you look closely at the plague doctor's clothes and equipment, it gives clues as to what people thought caused the plague.

- The doctor is wearing a hat, very thick clothes gloves and boots to avoid direct contact with the plague victims or their belongings.
- The nose cone is full of sweet-smelling herbs to ward off bad air.
- An **amulet** (jewellery) to ward off evil spirits is hidden under the sleeve of the coat.

Treatments: How did people try to treat the Great Plague?

- Doctors still had no cures for the plague. Physicians might have recommended bleeding or purging, but most physicians left London to save themselves from plague.
- People prayed for the sick or gave them magical or religious charms to wear.
- They cut open the buboes to let the pus out.
- A live chicken was strapped to a buboe in the hope that the illness would transfer to the chicken.
- Unqualified doctors sold 'Great Medicines' which they claimed had saved 'vast numbers' of lives. One such medicine, Theriac, or London Treacle, contained wine, herbs, spices, honey and opium.
- There were many different herbal remedies proposed. Some were a mixture of herbs and superstition. For example:
Wrap in woollen clothes, make the sick person sweat, which if he do, keep warm until the sores begin to rise. Then apply to the sores live pigeons cut in half or else a plaster made of yolk of an egg, honey, herb of grace and wheat flour.

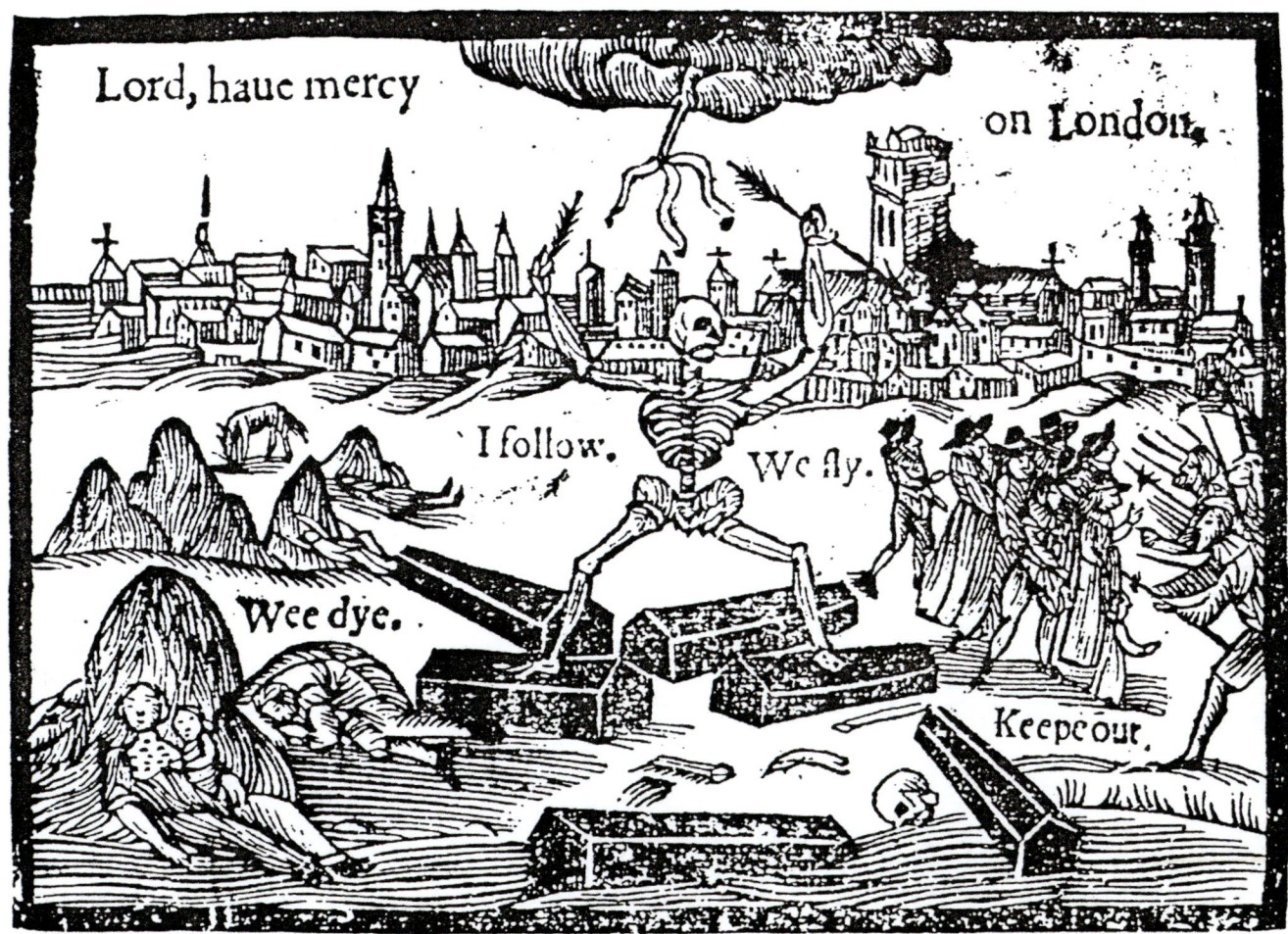

▲ **SOURCE L** A drawing from 1665 depicting the Great Plague. This drawing suggests that the only hope lies in God showing mercy

Prevention: How did people try to prevent the Great Plague from spreading?

As with the Black Death, the methods used to try to prevent the spread of the plague were closely linked to what people believed were the causes. People believed it was vital to keep the air sweet to ward off the bad air. They hung bunches of strong-smelling herbs (such as lavender or sage) in doorways and windows. They even carried bundles of herbs under their noses as they walked through the streets.

The Lord Mayor did his best to stop the plague spreading from infected houses.

- Victims were shut up in their homes and watchmen stood guard to stop anyone going in or out.
- When someone died, the body was examined by 'women searchers' to check that plague was the cause.
- Bedding had to be hung in the smoke of fires before it was used again.
- Fires were lit in the streets to cleanse the air of poisons.

Other regulations showed that people were making a connection between dirt and disease, even if they could not explain the link scientifically.

- Householders were ordered to sweep the street outside their doors.
- Pigs, dogs and cats were not to be kept inside the city. Stray dogs and cats were killed.
- Plays, bear-baitings and games were banned to prevent the assembly of large crowds.

However, these measures did not really work because:

- Parliament refused to turn the orders into laws because MPs refused to be shut in their houses.
- The King and his council left London. They discussed what to do about plague three times in seven months, but two of those discussions were about the King's safety.
- Nine men were put in charge of dealing with plague in London. Six of them left London as soon as they could.
- Plague symptoms were not reported. In fact, over 20 watchmen were murdered by people escaping from houses that had been shut up.
- Not enough men could be found to work as watchmen.
- Some watchmen and women searchers took the chance to steal from the sick.

Impact: The consequences of the Great Plague

The methods introduced in London by the Lord Mayor helped a little, but over a quarter of the population of London died in the Great Plague of 1665.

It took a combination of cold weather and then the Great Fire of London in 1666 to put an end to the Great Plague.

Following the Great Fire, central London was completely rebuilt. Narrow streets and wooden buildings were replaced by stone and brick buildings, and wider, better-paved streets.

For a time, London was healthier, but as the city became more and more crowded again during the Industrial Revolution, the benefits of the rebuilding disappeared.

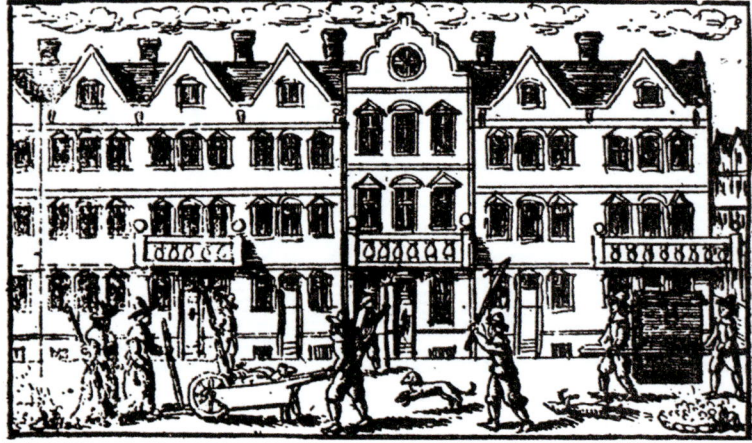

◀ **SOURCE M** A seventeenth-century print of a London street during the plague. It shows some of the plague orders being implemented. How many can you spot?

Part 2 Medical Renaissance period review

Review 1

Themes

1. The period summary chart below summarises the Medical Renaissance period. Study it carefully, then create a blank copy (with only the themes listed on the left-hand side) and try to complete the evidence of continuity and change columns **from memory alone**.
2. Review your attempt against the chart below and fill in any gaps using a **different coloured pen**. This will remind you what you are struggling to remember.

Period summary, c1500–c1700: The Medical Renaissance in England		
Theme	**Evidence of continuity**	**Evidence of change**
Ideas about the cause of disease and illness	Religious beliefs were still strong The imbalance of the four humours was still seen as a cause Bad air (miasma) was still considered a cause	Some people were beginning to make the connection between dirt and disease (see ways people tried to prevent the spread of the Great Plague)
Approaches to prevention	Cleanliness was promoted to prevent bad air (miasma) Quarantine was used during the Great Plague Governments did little to improve public health or stop diseases from spreading	There were some attempts by the Lord Mayor of London to prevent the spread of the Plague (1665)
Approaches to treatment	Bleeding and purging were still used Herbal remedies were still used Cures were still based on superstition Prayer was still used	More herbs from overseas (e.g. quinine for malaria) were used Chemical cures were used Transference was used
Care of the sick	The same people offered treatment – physicians, apothecaries, barber surgeons Hospitals still did not deal with infectious diseases Pest houses continued to treat those with infectious diseases, such as leprosy Most medical care was still provided by women within the family	Hospitals were set up and run by charities and local councils (e.g. St Bartholomew's in London)
Medical training		Training began to change Dissection was encouraged New ideas were published using the printing press New ideas were shared by The Royal Society

Review 2

What factors helped and hindered the Medical Renaissance in the years c1500 to c1700?

Complete a copy of the table below using the information in Part 2:

Factor	How it helped	How it hindered
Individuals	Thomas Sydenham encouraged doctors to examine a patient carefully before diagnosing illness. Sydenham discovered that measles and scarlet fever were different diseases. Sydenham encouraged others to ask questions and challenge the ideas of Galen. Sydenham's findings were published in 'Observationes Medicae' in 1676.	
Institutions: Church		
Institutions: Government		
Science and technology		
Attitudes in society		

Apply ▶ Exam Practice

Question 3 style

Explain **one** way in which medical training in medieval England was different from medical training in the Medical Renaissance. (4 marks)

Exam Tip

Comparing time periods (Question 3)

Look again at the advice on how to approach this type of question on page 39.

Remember to focus on explaining a similarity/difference and supporting your explanation with an example from both time periods.

- Think about the role of the Church.
- Think about the work of Thomas Sydenham and William Harvey.

Medical Renaissance exam practice

Exam Tip

Making a judgement (Question 5/6)

Your exam will include a question that asks you to make a judgement about how far you agree with a statement about causation, consequence, change, continuity or significance.

Remember to use the **3Ds**:

- **Decode** the question (work out the focus of the question).
- **Decide** how to organise your answer into paragraphs.
- **Develop** your answer by explaining and supporting the points you make.

What are the command words?
The question asks, 'how far do you agree?'. You need to try to agree and disagree with the statement before reaching a judgement.

What is the content focus?
Focus on William Harvey's discovery. Weigh this against other changes and developments during the Medical Renaissance in England. You need to include at least three aspects of knowledge throughout your answer.

> 'The **discovery made by William Harvey** was the **key turning point** in medicine in the years c1500 to c1700.'
> **How far do you agree?** Explain your answer.
> **(16 marks)**
> You may use the following in your answer:
> - Circulation of the blood
> - Galen
>
> You **must** also use information of your own.

How many marks are available?
'16 marks' indicates you should spend about 24 minutes on the question. You should try to write at least three paragraphs: at least one paragraph that agrees with the statement, at least one that disagrees and a conclusion. There are also 4 marks for SPAG. This means your spelling, punctuation and grammar. Check that you have used capital letters, commas, full stops and paragraphs correctly.

What is the conceptual focus?
The conceptual focus is significance. Describing the discovery made by William Harvey is not enough to get the higher-level marks. Focus on explaining why you agree and disagree that the discovery influenced medicine during the years c1500 to c1700 and then support this with examples from your knowledge.

Exam Tip

Use connectives and evidence for stronger arguments

When explaining why you agree and disagree with the statement, you have to prove your argument. For example:

William Harvey's discovery of the circulation of the blood was a turning point in medicine because he demonstrated the significance of a scientific approach. For example, Harvey dissected cold-blooded animals, such as frogs, because their heartbeat is slower. This meant that Harvey was able to see every muscle move and pump the blood. He also dissected human beings to gain a detailed knowledge of the heart. This led to Harvey proving that blood flowed in one direction as he was unable to pump liquid past the valves in the veins. Harvey also calculated the amount of blood inside a human body, and this resulted in him being able to show that the same blood was pumped around the body by the heart. The detailed nature of William Harvey's experiments in his discovery of the circulation of the blood demonstrates the significance of the scientific approach to medicine in the years c1500 to c1700. This approach enabled Harvey to disprove the traditional, and incorrect, ideas while encouraging others to challenge further using the same approach.

Use connectives to tie what you know to the statement

Phrases like 'this meant that', 'this led to' and 'this resulted in' are called connectives because they tie what you know to the statement and so help you prove your argument.

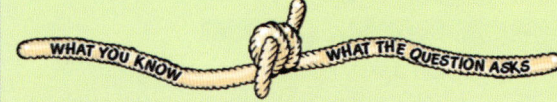

Add specific knowledge

Provide evidence to substantiate (support) your argument. Use phrases such as 'for example', 'such as' and 'this demonstrates' to introduce or flag your supporting evidence.

Apply ▶ Exam Practice

Question 5/6 style

Use the Exam Tip below to complete two developed explanations.

1. The first explanation should agree that the discovery by William Harvey was a turning point in medicine because it changed medical training about the human body. You can base that on what you have read on pages 42–43.
2. The second explanation should disagree and state that there were other developments that had a more significant impact on medicine in the years c1500 to c1700, such as The Royal Society. You can base this on what you learned on pages 34–35.

Exam Tip

Making a judgement (Question 5/6)

In the exam, you must make a judgement about how far you agree with the statement. The easiest way to do this is to write a conclusion at the end of your answer. The best answers will have their overall judgement running throughout the answer. For example, when answering the question in the Exam Practice box on page 51:

- Decide whether you agree or disagree that the discovery by William Harvey was the key turning point in medicine in the years c1500 to c1700. You could then begin your paragraph with:
 'In conclusion, William Harvey's discovery was a turning point but was not the key turning point in the years c1500 to c1700 …'
- Go on to explain why you have reached this judgement. You could argue that:
 '… the emergence of the printing press was the key turning point because it allowed new knowledge to be shared more widely and encouraged further developments in medicine.'

Apply ▶ Exam Practice

Question 5/6 style

'There was little progress in approaches to the prevention and treatment of disease and illness in the years c1250 to c1700.'

How far do you agree? Explain your answer. (16 marks)

You may use the following in your answer:

- Bloodletting
- The Great Plague in London, 1665

You **must** also use information of your own.

Part 3 Ideas about the cause of disease and illness c1700–c1900

Connect & Engage – Louis Pasteur

Louis Pasteur was born in France and was a university scientist, not a doctor. He was also a hugely determined man who made one of the most important breakthroughs in our understanding of disease.

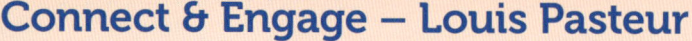

How did Louis Pasteur develop the Germ Theory?

Pasteur was asked to investigate why alcoholic drinks sometimes went sour. This was costing the French beer and wine industry a lot of money. Pasteur's solution was to heat the drinks briefly to kill off disease-causing bacteria. This process became known as **pasteurisation** and was also used to stop diseases such as tuberculosis being spread through contaminated milk.

As a result of this research, Pasteur became convinced that it was germs from the air that were causing the liquids to go sour. He also speculated that, in the same way, germs might be getting into humans and perhaps be causing disease.

How did Pasteur prove that the Germ Theory was correct?

Pasteur published his 'Germ Theory' in 1861. The French government paid for Pasteur to hire research assistants and set up a new laboratory where he could carry out experiments to try to prove that his Germ Theory was correct.

In 1865, he was called in to help the silk industry. A disease was killing the silkworms. He proved that the disease was being spread by germs in the air. This was the first time it was proved that germs were causing disease in animals.

Pasteur also started to investigate human diseases. However, he struggled to identify the specific bacteria that caused individual diseases.

> **Connect & Engage**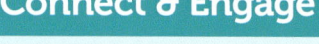
>
> **What was the impact of the Germ Theory?**
>
> Read both pages and explain why the Germ Theory was a turning point in the history of medicine.

How did others build on Pasteur's work?

Not everyone accepted Pasteur's findings, but some pioneers did – notably a German doctor named Robert Koch. In 1876, he and his research team made an important breakthrough. They found the bacterium that was causing anthrax (a disease that affected animals and humans). This was the first time anyone had identified the specific microbe that causes a particular disease.

Over the next 20 years, Koch and other scientists identified more bacteria causing individual diseases and this led to the development of **vaccines** to prevent them.

This finally persuaded people that bad air was not the cause of disease. For the first time, doctors understood what really did cause diseases and this revolutionised medicine in different ways. The diagram on the opposite page sums this up.

The significance of Pasteur and the Germ Theory

Before Pasteur

Miasma Theory of disease
By 1800, the main explanation of disease was **bad air** (**miasma**). This old idea made even more sense in the mid-1800s when towns were more crowded and filthy than ever before and were also more disease ridden.

Spontaneous generation
In the nineteenth century, using microscopes, scientists could see that rubbish was covered with bacteria. They could see germs on everything! The popular theory was that decaying matter was **creating these bacteria**. This was the theory of spontaneous generation.

Pasteur's ideas

Pasteur's Germ Theory argued that:
- Bacteria were not created by decaying matter, the bacteria **caused** the decay. Pasteur therefore challenged the theory of spontaneous generation.
- Germs got into the decaying matter from the air as germs were literally all around us all the time.
- Germs could cause wine or milk to go bad. They also got into humans and caused disease.

It was only a theory – it had to be proved and that took time.
And, though Pasteur made the breakthrough, others turned it into lifesaving treatments.

Short-term impact

- Robert Koch was the first to link an individual bacterium to an individual disease.
- Once specific bacteria had been linked to specific diseases, vaccines were developed to prevent them.
- Joseph Lister used **carbolic spray** to perform the first **antiseptic surgery**.

Summarise

Draw your own version of this memory aid, then add your own examples to support each consequence.

Germ Theory made a **VAST** difference:

Vaccinations developed, for example …
Acts to improve public health, for example …
Surgery became safer, for example …
Treatments improved, for example …

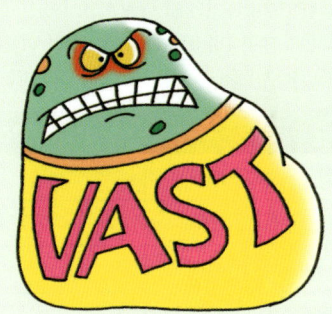

Long-term impact

New treatments: in the late 1800s, scientists developed the first chemical drugs (for example, **sulphonamides**) and, in the 1930s, the first **antibiotic** (for example, **penicillin**) that killed bacteria in the body was discovered.

Aseptic surgery: developed in the late nineteenth century. The aim was to make sure that operating theatres were germ free.

Improved public health: Pasteur's discovery encouraged councils and government to build sewers, to keep streets clean and to provide clean water.

Continuity and change in explanations of the cause of disease and illness

Research & Record

Explain why there was progress in the understanding of the cause of disease and illness in the nineteenth century.

Copy and complete the table below using the information on these pages and on pages 54–55.

Think carefully about the language you use to state how important each reason was. In column 2, choose a word or phrase from the scale on the right to show the level of importance. Do not fill in column 3 if you think a reason had no or only minimal impact.

Essential	No change could have happened without it
Important	Without it, change might have been less widespread or significant
Minimal	Had only a little impact
No importance	No influence at all

Reason	Importance	Explanation
The work of individuals		
The role of the Church		
The role of government		
Developments in science and technology		
Changes in attitudes in society		

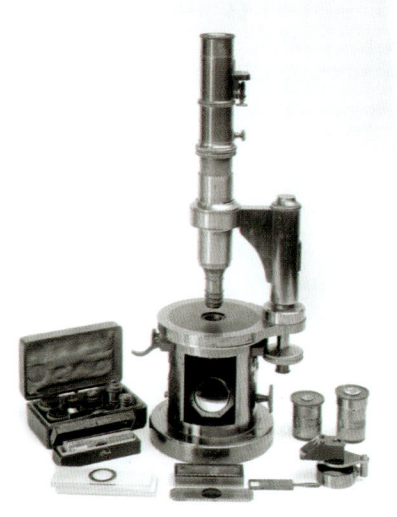

▲ **SOURCE A** A microscope from 1859

Old and new ideas

The eighteenth century saw change in the ideas about the cause of disease and illness. People no longer believed that God was in control of all events and so he was no longer thought to be the cause of disease and illness. People had moved away from believing in the Theory of the Four Humours too. People did still believe in miasma, but this theory was becoming less popular.

As you have seen on page 55, one new theory that did develop in the eighteenth century was spontaneous generation. Improvements in technology led to stronger microscopes. For the first time, scientists could see microbes and could see that they were present on decaying material such as vegetables and animals. The Theory of Spontaneous Generation was that the decaying material produced these microbes, rather than the microbes being the cause of the decay. Throughout the eighteenth century, this remained a theory as scientists were unable to prove that this was correct.

It was not until Louis Pasteur discovered germs (see pages 54–55) in the nineteenth century that there was a major change in the understanding of the cause of disease and illness.

Koch's work on microbes

Robert Koch was a German doctor. He developed Louis Pasteur's Germ Theory. Pasteur had identified that microbes were the cause of decay, but it was Robert Koch who successfully identified that different germs cause many different diseases.

Koch was just as ambitious as Pasteur and just as brilliant at detailed, painstaking work in his laboratory which was carried out with a team of assistants. The two men saw each other as rivals, especially after the war between France and Germany in 1870–71, which was won by Germany. Both men wanted to be successful to bring glory to their country.

> **Breakthrough 1: Linking bacteria to specific diseases**
>
> Koch investigated anthrax, a disease affecting animals, and discovered the **specific bacterium** that causes the disease. This was the first time anyone had identified a specific germ that caused a particular disease. It was also the long-awaited final proof that Pasteur's Germ Theory was correct.

> **Breakthrough 2: Making it easier to study bacteria**
>
> Koch then developed a method of **staining bacteria** to make them easier to study. They could be photographed using a new, high-quality photographic lens.
>
> Other scientists copied Koch's methods to discover bacteria that caused other diseases.

> **Breakthrough 3: Studying human disease**
>
> Pasteur used Koch's findings to develop a vaccine against anthrax (see page 54). Koch decided to get ahead again by becoming the first person to discover the specific germ that causes a human disease. He investigated the deadly disease of tuberculosis (TB). The TB bacterium was so small that it had been missed by other scientists so far, but Koch found a way of staining even such a tiny bacterium so that it stood out from other bacteria and human tissue.
>
> This was the major breakthrough he had been searching for. His research team followed this up by discovering the specific bacterium that causes **cholera** (another feared disease).

The significance of Robert Koch

- Koch's work encouraged other scientists to continue the search for specific microbes. In the last decades of the nineteenth century, scientists went on to identify the microbes that caused diphtheria, pneumonia, meningitis, plague and **dysentery**.
- Identifying the specific microbe for a disease was an enormous breakthrough. Now doctors knew they had to study the microbe to understand the symptoms of a disease. This led scientists to look for a way to remove the microbe in order to attack the disease.
- As with other discoveries, the spread of the ideas was as important as the discovery itself in terms of affecting the way doctors worked. Koch published his works and spoke at conferences to raise awareness of his discoveries. Koch was awarded a Nobel Prize for his work in 1905.

The impact of the Germ Theory in Britain

Once the cause of disease was understood and the individual microbes for specific diseases were starting to be identified, real progress could be made in medicine. As you will see in the next section, these discoveries allowed for progress in the prevention of disease and illness because vaccines could be developed.

Part 3 Approaches to treatment c1700–c1900

Improvements in hospital care and the influence of Nightingale on nursing and hospitals in Britain

> **Research & Record**
>
> **What changes did Florence Nightingale influence in hospitals?**
>
> Use pages 58–59 to complete your own copy of a table like this. Record examples of the influence of Florence Nightingale linked to nursing and hospital design.
>
> | Influence on nursing | Influence on hospitals |
> |---|---|
> | | |

Hospitals in the early 1800s were unsafe. In 1801, it was believed that there were only 3000 patients in hospitals. In 1851, the figure was still only 7619, according to the census. A major reason for this was the appalling death rate due to infection and the spread of disease. Even in 1861 the campaigner Florence Nightingale believed that 90 per cent of patients in London hospitals died. Most patients in hospital were elderly or poor. Anyone who had enough money would generally choose to be treated at home.

Florence Nightingale

Florence Nightingale had always wanted to be a nurse. She trained in Germany because she could not train in Britain. After her training, she worked as a nurse in a London hospital. In 1854, the Crimean War broke out between Britain, France and Russia. Nightingale was asked to go out to take care of the soldiers in the Crimea. She agreed and took 38 nurses with her.

At the main army hospital in Scutari, Nightingale set to work looking after the soldiers. However, she was appalled by the dirty conditions. She cleaned the hospital and the patients. She opened windows, regularly changed the bedding, provided good meals and had part of the ward rebuilt. These changes were so effective that the death rate fell from 40 to 2 per cent. Nightingale shared her approach and impact with the British government.

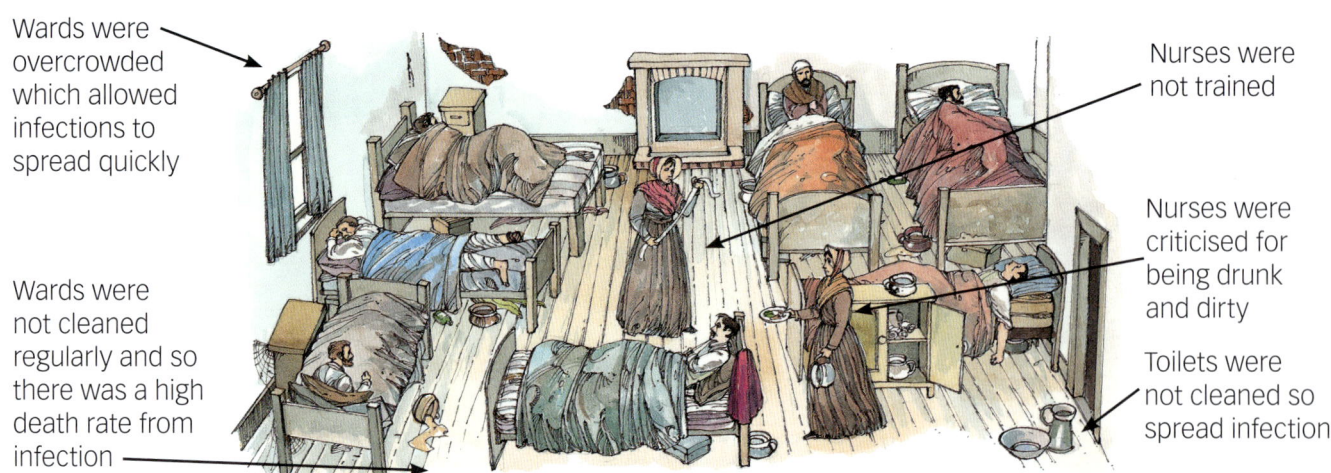

▲ **SOURCE B** A reconstruction drawing of a hospital ward around 1800

Labels:
- Wards were overcrowded which allowed infections to spread quickly
- Wards were not cleaned regularly and so there was a high death rate from infection
- Nurses were not trained
- Nurses were criticised for being drunk and dirty
- Toilets were not cleaned so spread infection

The influence of Nightingale: Nursing

When Florence Nightingale returned from the Crimea, she worked with the British government to improve hospital care. Florence Nightingale improved the care of patients by focusing on the training of nurses and the conditions in hospitals. In 1859, she wrote a book called *Notes on Nursing*. Nursing became a respected profession in which women were trained. In 1860, Nightingale opened her first Nightingale Training School for Nurses.

Her ideas were used to train nurses across Britain. Nurses were trained in the principles of cleanliness. They were also trained to change dressings and to be proper assistants to doctors and surgeons. Nightingale nurses were a separate but important new branch of the medical profession. Rather than being minders or cleaners they were an important part of the process of treatment.

Interestingly, Nightingale believed in the Miasma Theory. Even after Pasteur had discovered germs, she continued to believe that bad air was the main cause of disease and illness. She had always associated disease with dirt. Nightingale did not let doctors teach her nurses about Germ Theory because she felt that this would stop the nurses from focusing on keeping the hospital wards and patients clean.

The influence of Nightingale: Hospitals in the nineteenth century

In 1863 Nightingale wrote a book called *Notes on Hospitals*. This book was very influential and led to improvements in hospital design. The main changes that she influenced were:

- Cleanliness in hospitals was improved by providing clean water, good drains and sewers, and improved toilets.
- Ventilation in hospitals was improved by building more windows and having larger rooms to ensure patients breathed in clean air.
- Clothing, washing facilities and food for patients in hospitals were all improved.

Throughout the nineteenth century the wealthy and middle classes continued to be treated at home because this was believed to be healthier than going to a hospital ward. Nightingale was determined to change this situation and to make hospitals better and safer places for the sick. She set out her ideas in what became known as 'The Nightingale Principles'.

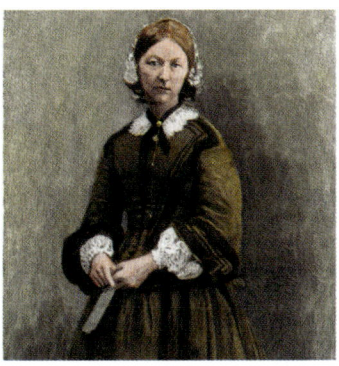

▲ A portrait of Florence Nightingale (1820–1910)

In my experience the main defects with hospitals are:
1. A large number of sick under the same roof, closely packed together
2. Lack of space
3. Lack of ventilation
4. Lack of light

The buildings themselves should avoid the following:
1. Defective means of natural ventilation and warming
2. Defective height of wards
3. Excessive width of wards between opposite windows
4. Having more than two rows of beds between the opposite windows
5. Arranging the beds along the dead walls
6. Having windows only on one side, or having a closed corridor connecting the wards
7. Absorbent materials for walls and ceilings
8. Defective water closets
9. Defective ward furniture
10. Defective accommodation for nurses and discipline
11. Defective kitchens
12. Defective laundries
13. Selection of bad sites and bad local climates
14. Erecting hospitals in towns
15. Defective sewerage
16. Construction without free circulation of external air

▲ **SOURCE C** Extracts from Florence Nightingale's *Principles*

The problems in surgery in the eighteenth century

Research & Record

What were the main problems facing surgeons in the early 1800s?

1. Look at Source D. Fill in a table like this. How is each problem shown in the source?
2. Read page 61. Why did these anaesthetics not fully solve the problem of pain?

	Clues that suggest this in the source
Surgeons were not respected. They were seen as butchers or torturers.	
Procedures were painful for the patient due to lack of effective anaesthetics.	
Infection could spread easily due to lack of effective antiseptics, and a crowded, unclean operating environment.	
There was very basic technology, surgery tools and equipment.	
Death rates were high (patients died from the shock of pain, blood loss and infection).	

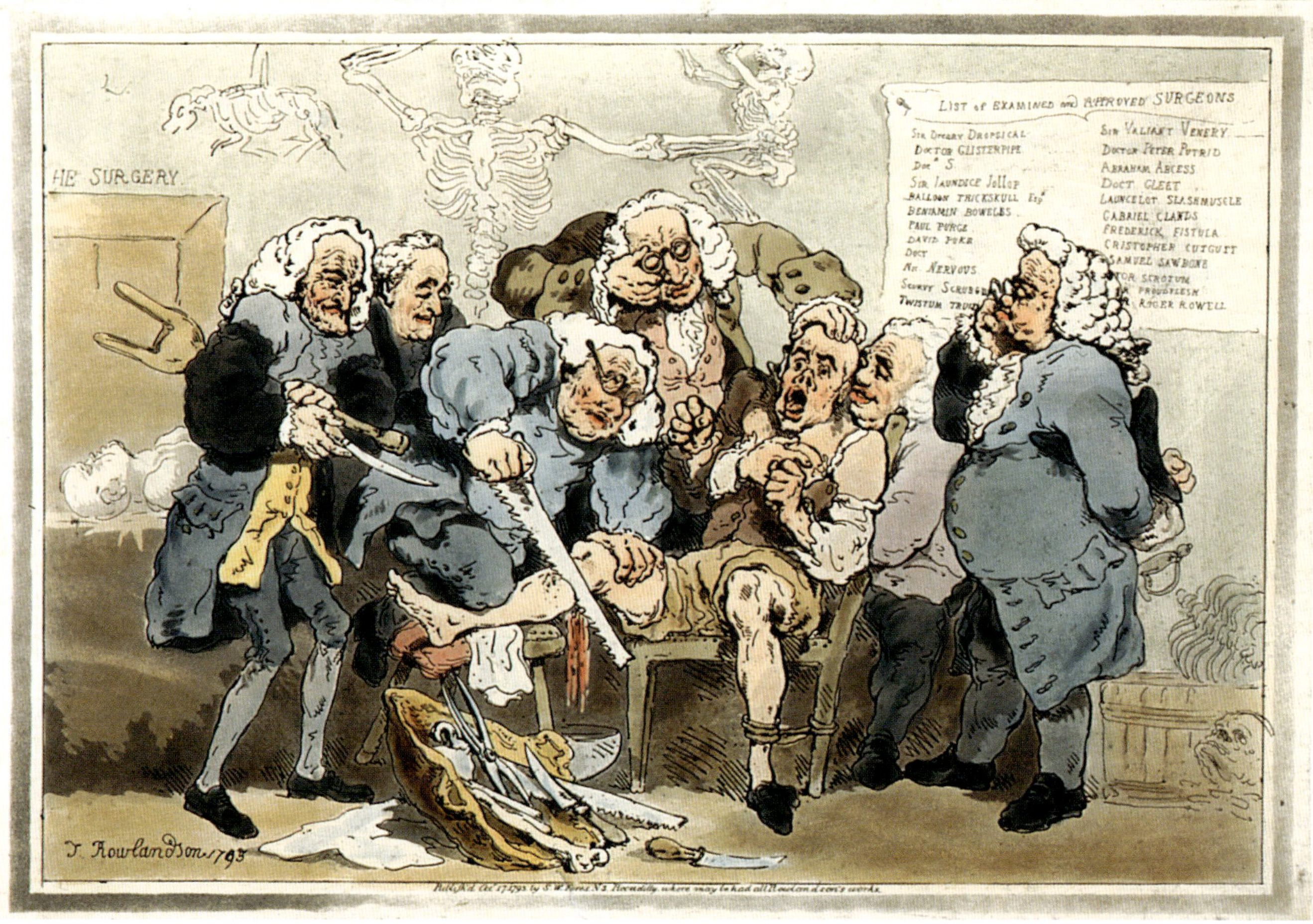

▲ **SOURCE D** A cartoon showing an amputation, published in 1793

Early anaesthetics

Through the centuries, surgeons tried various methods to deal with pain.

- In the Middle Ages, they used herbs such as mandrake and hemlock. Both could kill if too much was used.
- In the Renaissance period, they tried alcohol and opium. However, alcohol did not make the patient totally unconscious and opium could kill through overdose.

Speed

As nothing was totally effective, the only way to reduce pain was speed. The patient was held or tied down by the surgeon's assistants while the surgeon operated as quickly as possible. At the Battle of Borodino in 1812, Napoleon's surgeon, Dubois, is said to have amputated 200 limbs in 24 hours. Surgeons prided themselves on their speed. Speed was one sign of a good surgeon.

The danger of speed!

Speed could also cause problems. Robert Liston, a famous London surgeon, once amputated a leg in two-and-a-half minutes but worked so fast that he accidentally cut off his patient's testicles as well.

During another high-speed operation, Liston amputated the fingers of his assistant and slashed the coat of a spectator who, fearing that he had been stabbed, dropped dead with fright. And both the assistant and the patient died of infection after the operation.

Improved anaesthetics

The late 1700s and 1800s saw an explosion of interest in chemistry. Scientists studied the properties of different chemicals. They also found out that some chemicals could have effects on the human body. This resulted in improved anaesthetics.

Laughing gas

In 1799, Sir Humphry Davy discovered that 'laughing gas' (properly called nitrous oxide) reduced the sensation of pain. He suggested that it might be useful in surgery or dentistry. However, it did not make patients completely unconscious. Also, when an American dentist, Horace Wells, used it in a public demonstration, his patient was in agony. This damaged confidence in laughing gas as an anaesthetic.

Ether

In 1846, ether was used as an anaesthetic in an operation in America to remove a neck tumour. A year later, in 1847, ether was used by Robert Liston in London to anaesthetise a patient during a leg amputation. Ether worked better than anything else so far. However, ether also had drawbacks:

- It was difficult to inhale.
- It irritated the eyes and lungs, causing coughing and sickness.
- It could catch fire if exposed to a flame.
- It had a vile smell that took ages to go away.
- It was stored in large, heavy bottles so was difficult to carry around.

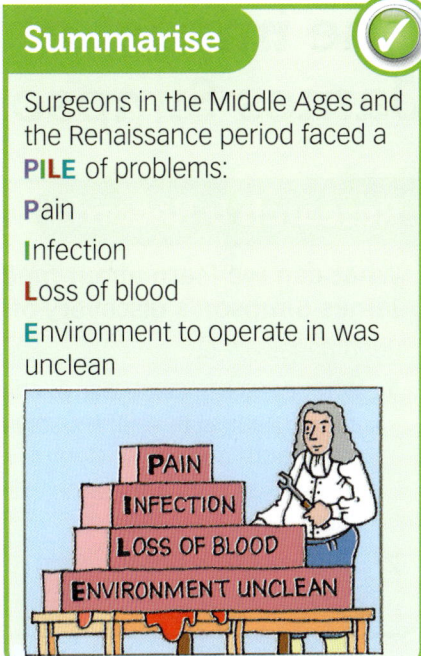

Summarise

Surgeons in the Middle Ages and the Renaissance period faced a **PILE** of problems:

Pain
Infection
Loss of blood
Environment to operate in was unclean

The impact of anaesthetics on surgery: James Simpson and chloroform

> **Research & Record**
>
> **What can we learn about medical developments in the years c1700 to c1900 from James Simpson's discovery of chloroform?**
>
> Read pages 62–63.
>
> 1 What does the discovery of chloroform tell us about medical developments in the eighteenth and nineteenth centuries? Copy and complete the table, giving examples from James Simpson's discovery of chloroform.
> 2 Why was there opposition to the use of chloroform in surgery?
>
> | | Example |
> |---|---|
> | The role of the individual | |
> | The scientific approach | |
> | The role of technology | |
> | Attitudes in society | |

The discovery of chloroform

James Simpson was Professor of Midwifery at Edinburgh University. He had used ether as a painkiller but was searching for a better anaesthetic. One evening in 1847, he and several colleagues sat around a table experimenting with different chemicals to see what anaesthetic effects they had. Simpson wrote later:

Simpson realised that he had discovered a very effective anaesthetic. Chloroform was faster-acting and gentler than ether. Within days, he started using it to help women in childbirth and in other operations. He wrote articles about his discovery and other surgeons started to use it in their operations.

> ▼ **SOURCE E**
>
> I poured some of the chloroform fluid into tumblers in front of my assistants, Dr Keith and Dr Duncan, and myself. Before sitting down to supper, we all inhaled the fluid, and were all 'under the table' in a minute or two, to my wife's consternation and alarm.

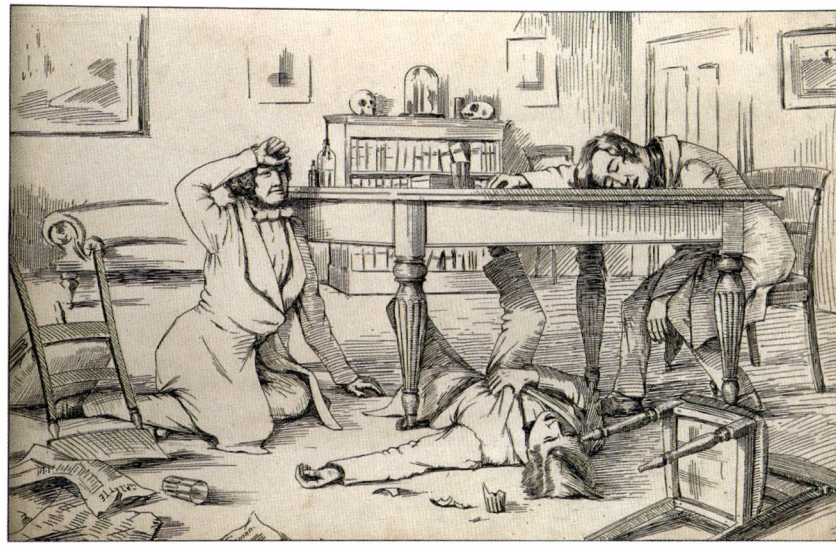

◀ **SOURCE F** Simpson and friends recovering from the effects of chloroform. A drawing made in 1857. Simpson is on the left.

Opposition to chloroform

There was a lot of opposition to chloroform for several different reasons.

Reason 1: Chloroform was new and untested

No one knew if there would be long-term side effects on the bodies or minds of patients. They also did not know what dose to give to different patients.

When Hannah Greener died during a routine operation (see Source G) this scared surgeons and gave opponents of anaesthetics powerful evidence of the dangers of chloroform.

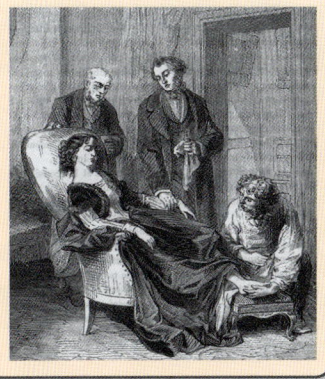

▶ **SOURCE G** This engraving shows the death of Hannah Greener in 1848. She died from an overdose of chloroform while she was having a toenail removed.

Reason 2: 'Pain is good'

Some people were opposed to the use of anaesthetics to ease pain on principle.

▼ **SOURCE H** Letter to the medical journal *The Lancet* in 1853:

> It is a most unnatural practice. The pain and sorrow of labour exert a most powerful and useful influence upon the religious and moral character of women and upon all their future relations in life.

▼ **SOURCE I** Letter to the medical journal *The Lancet* in 1849:

> The infliction [of pain] has been invented by the Almighty God. Pain may even be considered a blessing of the Gospel, and being blessed admits to being made either well or ill.

▼ **SOURCE J** A quotation from Army Chief of Medical Staff, 1854:

> … the smart use of the knife is a powerful stimulant and it is much better to hear a man bawl lustily than to see him sink silently into the grave.

Reason 3: It increased the risk of infection

Anaesthetics did not make surgery safer. With a patient asleep, doctors soon attempted more complex operations. They therefore carried infections deeper into the body and caused more loss of blood. The number of people dying from surgery increased from the 1850s to the early 1870s, which is known as surgery's 'Black Period'. In the 1870s, some surgeons stopped using chloroform because they were concerned about the high death rate (1 in 2500 operations). They returned to using ether mixed with nitrous oxide.

How was opposition overcome?

James Simpson played a leading role in promoting chloroform. He used it regularly and communicated to other doctors how it could be used safely.

Then, a breakthrough came when Queen Victoria was given chloroform during the delivery of her eighth child in 1853. She publicly praised 'that blessed chloroform'. With the support of the Queen, opposition to anaesthetics was doomed!

Consequences of chloroform

In the short term, developments in anaesthetics meant that more complex operations could be carried out. Surgeons could work more slowly and carefully without fear that their patients might die from shock. However, this also increased the risk of infection (described in Reason 3), so it was not a totally positive outcome.

In the longer term, the power of chloroform encouraged others to search for even better anaesthetics.

- Other chemicals were used which relaxed muscles as well as simply putting patients to sleep.
- Local anaesthetics were developed which numbed pain in one specific area of the body.

This took time, but Simpson's use of chloroform had been the turning point.

The impact of antiseptics on surgery: Lister and carbolic acid

Research & Record

How did Joseph Lister change surgery?
Use pages 64–65 to fill in a bingo card like the one below. It should help you collect evidence to:
- prove the significance of Lister's work
- identify the factors that helped Lister
- explain why Lister also faced opposition.

Lister bingo		
What new development had made surgery even more dangerous by 1860?	**By what percentage** did deaths from amputations fall when Lister used carbolic acid?	**How** was carbolic acid used before Lister used it as an antiseptic?
Give two examples of liquids used to keep wounds clean before Lister.	**Which two famous scientists** helped Lister's ideas become more widely accepted?	**Give two reasons** why Lister was partly to blame for the opposition he faced.
List three dangerous things that surgeons did before Lister changed surgery.	**List three examples** of how Lister improved his methods.	**List three reasons** why people opposed Lister's methods.

What was surgery like before Lister?

An operation without anaesthetics was horrible. Patients sometimes died just from the shock of the pain. However, many more patients died from something much less dramatic – infection after the operation.

Doctors knew infection could be fatal. They had used liquids such as wine and vinegar to keep wounds clean for centuries.

However, before Pasteur's Germ Theory, no one knew what was causing the infection, so surgeons did things that seem obviously dangerous to us today.

- They reused bandages, spreading **gangrene** and skin infections from patient to patient.
- They did not wash their hands before an operation.
- They did not **sterilise** their equipment.
- Some surgeons operated wearing old blood- and pus-stained clothes.

This was how they had done operations for years. It was what they were used to.

What inspired Lister to look for new ways to stop infection?

Joseph Lister was one of the outstanding surgeons of the nineteenth century. He was keenly interested in science and applying it to medicine. He had researched gangrene – trying to understand the way that infection spread.

Most importantly, he knew all about Pasteur's work on the Germ Theory. It was Pasteur's work that drove Lister to look for ways to kill bacteria in the wound.

His solution was carbolic acid.

Where did Lister's idea of using carbolic acid come from?

The idea to use carbolic acid came from sewage! In 1864, Lister observed how carbolic acid was used to reduce the smell of sewage that was used to fertilise the land. He noted how it also destroyed the parasites that usually infect cattle feeding on such land.

Lister experimented with carbolic acid to treat people with compound fractures (where the bone breaks through the skin). Infection often developed in these open wounds. Lister applied carbolic acid to the wound and used bandages soaked in it. He found that the wounds healed and did not develop gangrene.

What impact did Lister's work have in the short term?

Lister went on to use carbolic acid when he performed amputations. It dramatically reduced deaths from infection (see Source K). In 1867, Lister published his results, showing the value of using carbolic acid. He also worked at improving his method so that bacteria were being killed at every stage of an operation.

▼ **SOURCE K** From Lister's record of amputations

	Total amputations	Died	Percentage who died
1864–66 (without antiseptics)	35	16	45.7%
1867–70 (with antiseptics)	40	6	15.0%

Handwashing with carbolic before operations avoided the surgeon carrying infection into wounds.

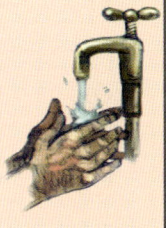

Carbolic spray killed germs in the air around the operating table.

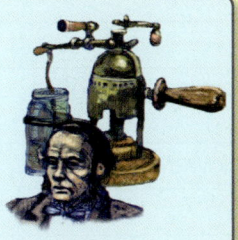

Tying up blood vessels with ligatures soaked in carbolic after surgery helped to prevent infection.

Why was there opposition to antiseptics?

It was unpleasant
Carbolic spray soaked the operating theatre. It cracked the surgeon's skin and made everything smell unpleasant.

Pasteur's ideas spread slowly
Even some trained surgeons found it hard to accept that tiny organisms were all around, causing disease. One surgeon joked with his assistants to shut the door of the operating room 'in case one of Mr Lister's microbes flew in'.

It slowed down operations
The new precautions caused extra work. Despite anaesthetics, surgeons still thought speed was essential – often because of the problem of bleeding.

Lister was not a showman
Unlike Pasteur, Lister did not give impressive public displays. In fact, he appeared cold and arrogant, and he criticised other surgeons. Many surgeons regarded him as a fanatic.

It did not always work
Some surgeons tried Lister's methods but did not achieve the same results. This was usually because they were less careful, but that did not stop them criticising Lister.

Lister changed his techniques
He tried other techniques because he wanted to find a substance that would work as well as carbolic spray, but without the corrosion that it caused. His critics said he was changing his methods because they did not work.

How was opposition overcome?

By Lister's determination

Lister's demonstrations and teachings helped to overcome opposition. In 1869, he became Professor of Clinical Surgery at Edinburgh University. Over the next eight years, he demonstrated his methods to over 1500 medical students. In 1877, he moved to King's College Hospital, London to train young surgeons.

With help from others

Then came a link to another great name in medical history. In 1878, Robert Koch discovered the bacterium which caused septicaemia (blood poisoning). This gave a great boost to Lister's ideas. By the end of the century, they were widely accepted.

Once the opposition was overcome, Lister's methods marked a turning point in surgery.

The extent of change in care and treatment

Research & Record

How had care and treatment in hospitals changed by 1900?

Look back and use information from pages 58–61, then use information on pages 66–67 to complete your own copy of this table.

Hospitals in the early 1800s	How this changed by 1900
Nurses were not trained	
Hospitals were not cleaned regularly	
Hospitals were overcrowded	
Patients were given a bed without consideration of their illness	
Hospitals were a place where the sick were cared for	
Surgery was painful for the patient	
Infections could spread easily in the operating theatres	
There was a high death rate as a result of surgery	

The period c1700–c1900 was a time of major change, but this did not mean that all aspects of medicine changed. On the whole, there was little to no change in the treatment of illness between 1700 and 1900. People still relied on herbal remedies. Some patients bought patent medicines known as cure-alls. These were pills that were claimed to cure everything from fever and tuberculosis to smallpox and measles. They were made from various substances including lard, wax, ginger, soap and aloe. However, as we have already seen with surgery, there was change in the care and treatment that people received in hospitals.

Hospitals

By 1900, hospitals looked very different from how they had looked in 1700. Hospitals were built with different wards to separate infectious patients. Operating theatres and specialist departments were being built. Cleanliness was a priority and, by 1900, the focus was on preventing germs from entering a hospital ward or operating room. Doctors and nurses received proper training. The role of a hospital had completely changed from being a place where the sick were cared for to a place where they were treated for disease and illness.

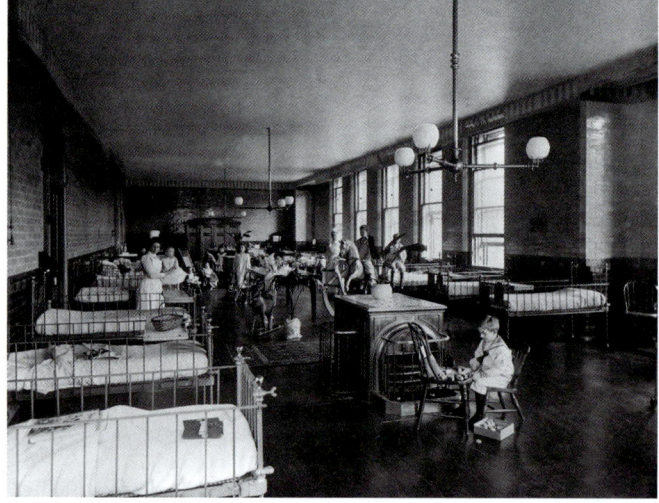

▲ **SOURCE L** A ward in Great Ormond Street Hospital, built in 1875

Connect & Engage

Where can you see evidence of the impact of Florence Nightingale in Source L?

Antiseptic surgery leads to aseptic surgery

The use of Lister's methods, which killed germs on the wound (see page 64), was called antiseptic surgery. By the late 1890s, this had developed into **aseptic surgery**, which meant removing all possible germs from the operating theatre. To ensure absolute cleanliness:

- Operating theatres and hospitals were carefully cleaned.
- All instruments were steam-sterilised.
- Surgeons no longer wore ordinary clothes but surgical gowns and face masks.
- Sterilised rubber gloves were introduced (see panel).

Surgery becomes more ambitious

With two of the basic problems of surgery now solved, surgeons attempted more ambitious operations.

- The first successful operation to remove an infected appendix came in the 1880s. Surgery on the small intestine, to stop the spread of cancer, also started around this time.
- The first heart operation was carried out in 1896, when surgeons repaired a heart damaged by a stab wound.

James Simpson and Joseph Lister had made major contributions. Their work helped make such operations possible. As surgeons started to perform more complex and safer operations, their status improved.

'A true glove story'

Caroline Hampton was an operating-theatre nurse. She developed a skin problem from the chemicals used to disinfect hands before operations. She showed her hands to William Halsted, a surgeon, and he arranged for the Goodyear Rubber Company (famous for car tyres) to make a pair of thin rubber gloves to protect Caroline's hands. Within a year, the nurse and the surgeon were married! And Halsted spread the idea of wearing rubber gloves during operations.

Summarise

1. Can you remember the four problems that surgeons faced in the early 1800s? What did PILE stand for? (Go back to page 61 if you can't remember.)

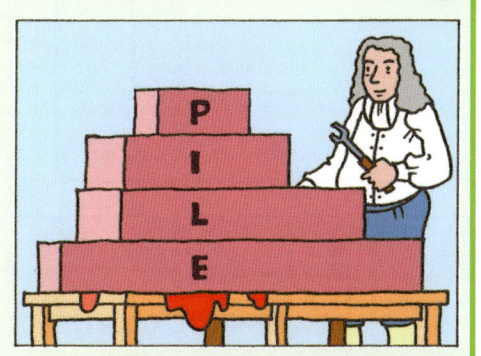

2. Explain how three of these problems had been tackled by 1900. Use this AAA memory aid to help you.

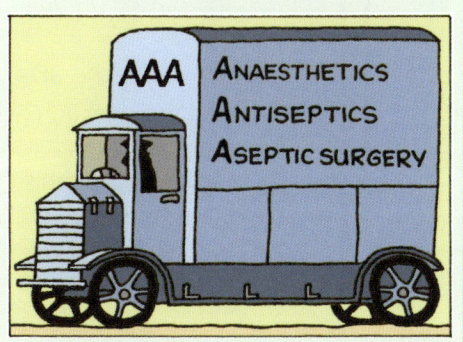

The extent of change in care and treatment exam practice

Apply ▶ Exam Practice

Question 3 style

Explain **one** way in which the care provided in hospitals in the years c1250 to c1500 was different from the care provided in hospitals in the years c1700 to c1900. (4 marks)

Look again at the advice on how to approach this type of question on page 39.

This question compares **one feature** (the care provided in hospitals) in two different time periods.
Focus on **difference**. Do not go into similarities.
When you compare the feature of hospital care in different periods, you need to support with an example from both time periods. • Consider who was admitted to hospital in both periods and what care they were given. • Consider who cared for the those in hospitals in both periods and what training they received.

Revision Tip

As you learn about and reflect on hospital care in Britain from c1250 to the present day, look for change and continuity. You can organise your notes into a table similar to this one:

Hospital care in Britain, c1250–present	
Examples of change	Examples of continuity

Think about why hospital care changed using the following factors:
- Individuals
- The role of the Church
- The role of government
- Science and technology
- Attitudes in society

Apply ▶ Exam Practice

Question 4 style

Explain why there were improvements in surgery in the years c1700 to c1900. (12 marks)

You may use the following in your answer:
- Chloroform
- Joseph Lister

You **must** also use information of your own.

Exam Tip

Explaining change or continuity (Question 4)

Look at the advice on page 45 on how to tackle this type of question and produce a high-level explanation.

Remember to use the **3Ds**:
- **Decode** the question (work out the focus of the question).
- **Decide** how to organise your answer into paragraphs.
- **Develop** your answer by explaining and supporting the points you make. Explain why there were improvements in surgery in the years c1700 to c1900. Support each reason with specific knowledge. Make sure you have included three aspects of knowledge across your whole answer.

Exam Tip

Use connectives and evidence for stronger arguments

When explaining why improvements in medicine took place, you have to prove the reason was a cause. For example:

There were improvements in surgery in the years c1700 to c1900 because of the commitment of key individuals. For example, James Simpson was a Professor of Midwifery and he was committed to easing the pain experienced by women in childbirth. While experimenting with different substances to find a more effective anaesthetic than ether, Simpson discovered the power of chloroform. He was knocked out very quickly after inhaling the substance. Simpson believed he had found an anaesthetic that was faster-acting and gentler. Simpson began using chloroform to help women in childbirth within days and other surgeons followed him after he shared his findings in medical articles. This demonstrates that the commitment of an individual, in this case James Simpson, was key to easing the problem of pain in surgery. Simpson wasn't happy using ether and this led to his search for a better anaesthetic. He also shared his experiences in medical journals, which resulted in other midwives and patients benefitting from chloroform to ease the problem of pain in surgery.

Add specific knowledge
Provide evidence to substantiate (support) your argument. Use phrases such as 'for example', 'such as' and 'this demonstrates' to introduce or flag your supporting evidence.

Use connectives to tie what you know to the question
Phrases like 'this meant that', 'this led to' and 'this resulted in' are called connectives because they tie what you know to the question and so help you to prove your argument.

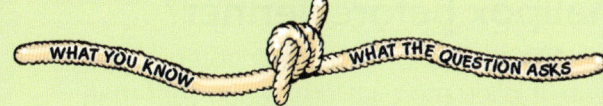

Apply ▶ Exam Practice

Question 4 style

Use the Exam Tip to complete two developed explanations.

- The second paragraph could prove that developments in scientific knowledge led to improvements in surgery.
- The third paragraph could prove that developments in technology led to improvements in surgery.

Part 3 Approaches to prevention c1700–c1900

Case study: Jenner and the development of vaccination

> **Research & Record**
>
> **Why was the work of Edward Jenner so significant?**
>
> To explain the significance of an individual you need to know three main things:
>
> 1. **The situation before** the individual made their discovery: what problems did people face?
> 2. **The impact at the time**: what changed as a result of their work in the short term?
> 3. **The long-term impact**: why was their work a turning point in medicine?
>
> Use pages 70–71 to make research notes under these three headings.

How did people try to prevent smallpox before Jenner?

In the 1700s, smallpox was as frightening as plague. It killed more children each year than any other disease and thousands of adults too. Survivors could be badly disfigured.

In China and Asia, a technique had been discovered to stop people catching smallpox. It was called **inoculation**. It involved spreading pus from a smallpox spot into a cut in the skin of a healthy person. If the person was lucky, they got only a mild dose of smallpox and did not catch it again because their body had developed a resistance to smallpox. During the eighteenth century, this method of prevention became popular in England.

However, there were dangers with inoculation:

- The person inoculated could get a severe dose of smallpox and die.
- The person inoculated could pass smallpox on to someone else.
- Most people could not afford inoculation so were not protected. Doctors could charge up to £20 per patient (£1500 in today's money).

How did Jenner make his discovery?

In the 1790s, Edward Jenner was an experienced doctor. He had studied under John Hunter, the greatest surgeon of the time. He kept in touch with Hunter when he began work as a country doctor in Gloucestershire in the 1770s. Hunter taught his students to observe patients carefully and to test their ideas through experimentation. Jenner followed Hunter's advice to discover a new way of preventing smallpox.

Like other country doctors, Jenner knew that milkmaids who caught cowpox, a mild disease, never got smallpox. In the 1790s, Jenner decided to carry out experiments to see if he could use cowpox to prevent smallpox in other people. He carefully recorded each experiment in detail.

In one famous experiment, Jenner took cowpox pus from a sore on the hand of Sarah Nelmes, a dairy maid. Jenner inserted the matter into a healthy eight-year-old boy called James Phipps. Jenner then inoculated the young boy with smallpox matter, but no disease followed. Several months later, Jenner again inoculated the boy with smallpox matter, but still no disease followed.

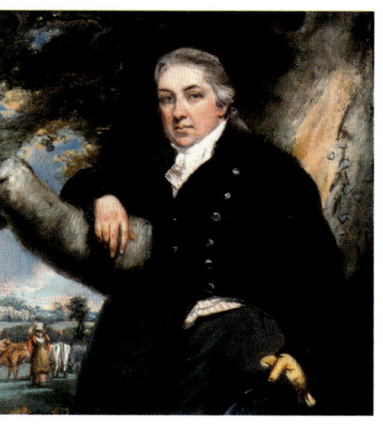

◀ A portrait of Edward Jenner (1749–1823)

What was the impact of Jenner's work at the time?

Jenner did 23 similar experiments. Then, in 1798, he felt sure enough of his method to publish his findings and show people how to use it. He called it vaccination (the Latin word for cow is *vacca*). Jenner's book also included his evidence that this really worked. In Britain, the government gave Jenner £30,000 to develop his work and vaccination became widely used. Deaths from smallpox fell quickly.

However, the government did not make vaccination compulsory until 1852, 50 years after Jenner's research. This was partly because there was opposition to Jenner's methods by groups such as the Anti-Vaccine Society (see diagram). It took time to convince people that his methods were safe and effective. Also, some people did not think that laws should be passed to make vaccination compulsory because the government should not interfere in people's lives.

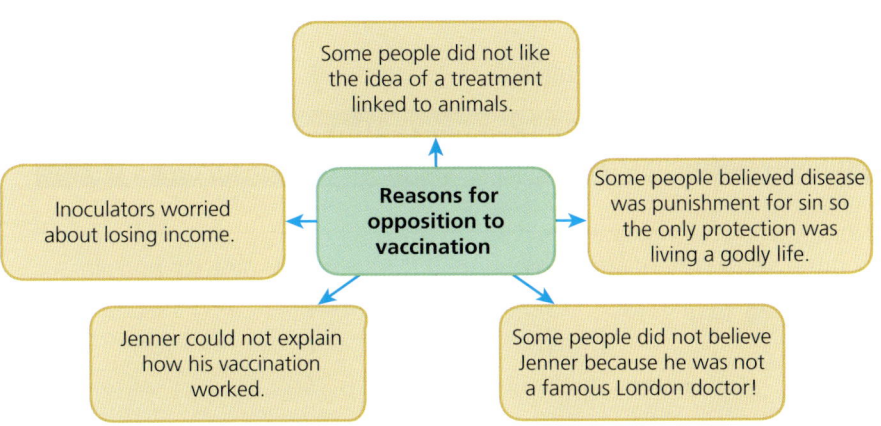

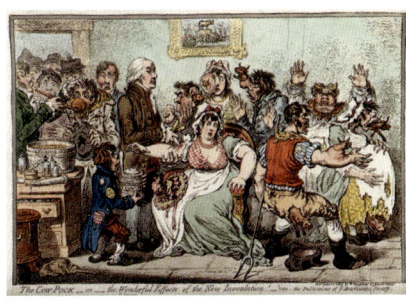

▲ **SOURCE M** A cartoon published by the Anti-Vaccine Society in 1802. Jenner is shown vaccinating a worried woman

Connect & Engage

1. What can you see happening in the cartoon?
2. How has the artist tried to convince people not to have the smallpox vaccine?

Why was Jenner's work important in the long term?

Smallpox was eradicated as a killer disease. Source N shows how deaths from smallpox fell in Britain. Vaccination was compulsory from 1852 but this was only strictly enforced from 1871 (after a major epidemic). Parents were fined for not having their children vaccinated. By the 1970s, smallpox had been wiped out worldwide.

Other scientists built on Jenner's work and developed vaccinations against other diseases. Jenner did not know why vaccination worked. Vaccination was a 'one-off' discovery, made because Jenner observed the connection between cowpox and smallpox. However, in the long term, after the discovery of the Germ Theory, other vaccines were developed which dramatically reduced deaths from infectious diseases (see page 72).

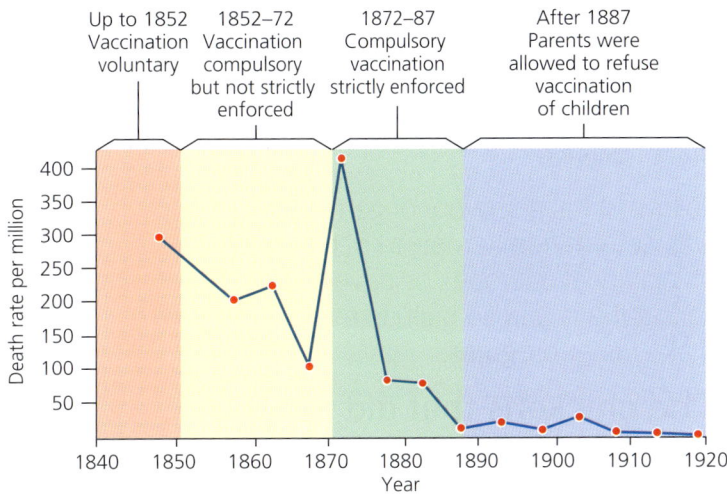

▲ **SOURCE N** Deaths from smallpox, 1840–1920

New approaches to prevention: The development and use of vaccinations

Research & Record

What impact did vaccinations have on ways of preventing the spread of disease and illness?

The development of the smallpox vaccine, the Germ Theory and the identification of bacteria that caused specific diseases led to improved ways of preventing disease. However, people did not benefit immediately from these changes.

1. Make a copy of the table below and use what you have learned about the smallpox vaccine and the Germ Theory on pages 70–71 to record the ways in which the prevention of disease and illness progressed quickly and ways in which prevention was slower to change.
2. Then, use the information on this page to add more to your table.

Evidence that change in the prevention of disease and illness happened quickly	Evidence that change in the prevention of disease and illness happened at a slower pace

3. Once your table is complete, evaluate the speed of change in preventing the spread of disease and illness following vaccinations. Choose the appropriate phrase from the scale below and explain why you have come to this conclusion.

A total change in … — Significant change — Some changes but mainly continuity — Considerable continuity — No change in …

4. Choose the strongest piece of evidence to support your overall conclusion.

Pasteur discovers new vaccinations

Once Pasteur had discovered germs (see page 54), medical professionals were able to explain why Jenner's smallpox vaccine was successful. It was understood that a weakened version of the disease led the body's immune system to produce antibodies that will fight a future stronger version of the disease.

Following his discovery of germs, Pasteur was determined to match Koch's discoveries of individual microbes by developing more vaccinations and so built up a research team to make faster progress.

The chickens that did not die

The team started work trying to help the farming industry because an epidemic of chicken cholera was killing many thousands of chickens. In 1880, Pasteur was working with his team, injecting chickens with the germ that caused chicken cholera so that they could then try to cure them of the disease. One of the team, Charles Chamberland, forgot to inject the chickens before the summer holiday, and on his return used the germs he should have used before the break. The chickens did not become ill, even when injected again – with some fresh germs.

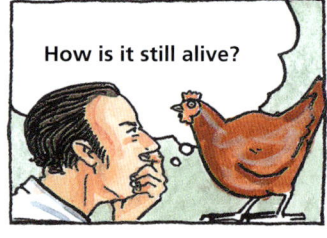

Pasteur solved the riddle of the chickens that did not die. He realised that the germs left over the summer had weakened and were not strong enough to kill the chickens, but instead they protected the chickens from a strong dose of cholera. When people said it had been a lucky discovery, he replied 'No! Chance only favours prepared minds.'

Anthrax vaccine

Now Pasteur could create other vaccines. At first, he continued to work on animals, producing a vaccine against anthrax. He tested this successfully in a public experiment and the news spread rapidly around Europe.

Rabies vaccine

After his success with vaccines against animal diseases, Pasteur turned to human diseases. He investigated rabies, testing his vaccine successfully on dogs, but did not know if it would work on people. The chance to find out came in 1885, when he tested his vaccine on Joseph Meister, a boy who had been bitten by a rabid dog. If the vaccine did not work, the boy would die. Pasteur gave Joseph 13 injections over a two-week period. Joseph survived.

Other scientists follow

Other scientists set to work finding vaccines that could prevent other human diseases. Their successes included vaccines against: typhoid (1896), tuberculosis (1906), diphtheria (1913), tetanus (1927), measles (1950s) and polio (1950s).

Summarise

Develop memory aids for the key individuals you have studied in the eighteenth and nineteenth centuries.

1. Can you remember the memory aid for Vesalius? (CLUE: It should be as easy as ABCDE). Check page 31 to see if you got it right.
2. Below is a memory aid for Jenner. Use key words and images to produce memory aids for Nightingale, Pasteur and Koch.

Jenner's discovery SAVED lives

Smallpox
Anti-Vaccine Society (opposed him)
Vaccination (from cowpox)
Experiments (for example, James Phipps)
Death rates fell

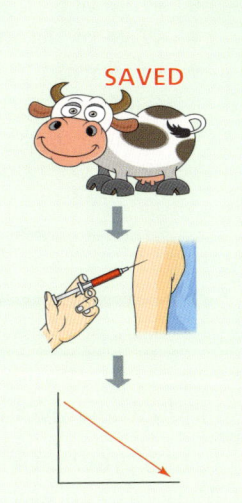

Exam Tip

Explaining change or continuity (Question 4)

Look at the advice on page 45 on how to tackle this type of question and produce a high-level explanation.

Remember to use the **3Ds**:

- **Decode** the question (work out the focus of the question).
- **Decide** how to organise your answer into paragraphs.
- **Develop** your answer by explaining and supporting the points you make. Explain why there were developments in the prevention of disease and illness in the years c1700 to c1900. Support each reason with specific knowledge. Make sure you have included three aspects of knowledge across your whole answer.

Apply — Exam Practice

Question 4 style

Explain why there were developments in the prevention of disease and illness in the years c1700 to c1900. (12 marks)

You may use the following in your answer:
- Germ Theory
- Vaccination

You **must** also use information of your own.

Part 3 Case study: Fighting cholera in London, 1854

> **Research & Record**
>
> **Why was the work of Dr John Snow important in the fight against cholera in London in 1854?**
>
> Read pages 74–76.
>
> 1 Answer the questions below about Dr John Snow's work on cholera in London in 1854:
>   - Why was cholera such a frightening disease?
>   - What methods were used to prevent cholera in the 1830s and 1840s?
>   - What was Dr John Snow's idea about the cause of cholera?
>   - What did Dr John Snow discover about the Broad Street pump?
>   - What was the government's reaction to Dr John Snow's discovery?
> 2 How far did the discovery made by Dr John Snow lead to changes in the fight against cholera in London in 1854? Make your decision using the continuum below and explain your decision fully.
>
> A total change in … — Significant change — Some changes but mainly continuity — Considerable continuity — No change in …

The Industrial Revolution caused the following conditions:

- Towns grew rapidly.
- As people moved to the towns for work, their population increased.
- Houses were built quickly and very close together.
- Water was provided by shared pipes and pumps in streets.
- Houses had to share outside toilets.

These conditions led to the spread of many diseases, such as typhus, diphtheria and scrofula. In the 1830s a terrifying new disease called cholera appeared in Britain and spread rapidly through the country, especially in the cities. Diseases like this were frightening because no one understood the cause or how to stop them.

Cholera epidemics

There were four major cholera epidemics between 1831 and 1865. Cholera was as terrifying as plague had been in previous centuries. It was caused by drinking unclean water. Violent sickness and diarrhoea led to severe dehydration and death. It could kill its victims in less than a day. The epidemic of 1848–49 killed 53,293 people. Cholera spread because germs from **cesspools** infected the water supply. But people did not know this. So, responses to cholera were a familiar mix of old and new, common sense and supernatural remedies (see panel).

Methods used to prevent the spread of cholera in the 1830s and 1840s

- To protect against bad air: burning barrels of tar; inhaling vinegar; smoking cigars
- Praying to God or wearing lucky charms
- Taking patent medicines that 'guaranteed' protection
- Burning the clothes and bedding of victims
- Quarantine – guards stopped poor people entering the city

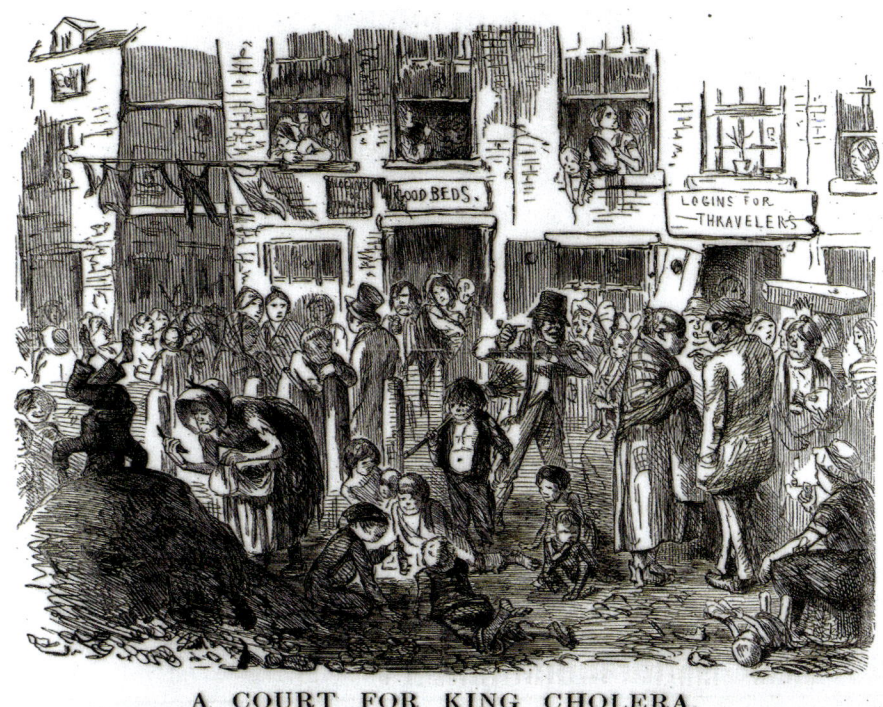

▲ **SOURCE O** A cartoon published in 1852 in Punch magazine. A court was an enclosed area of housing, often dark and over-populated

The significance of Dr John Snow and the Broad Street pump

John Snow was a doctor and surgeon. He was interested in the scientific approach to the observation of health issues. In 1849, he published a book putting forward his view that cholera spread through water, not in 'bad air'. His suggestion was mocked by many doctors.

The research

In 1854, another cholera outbreak gave him the chance to prove his theory right. Cholera had killed over 500 people around Broad Street in central London, near to Snow's surgery, in just ten days.

This led Snow to map out the deaths in detail. He linked all the deaths to a single water pump on Broad Street.

He found that a workhouse prison near Broad Street had virtually no cases of cholera because it had its own well. In contrast, Snow discovered that a lady from another part of London had died from cholera because she enjoyed the Broad Street water so much that she had it delivered to her home.

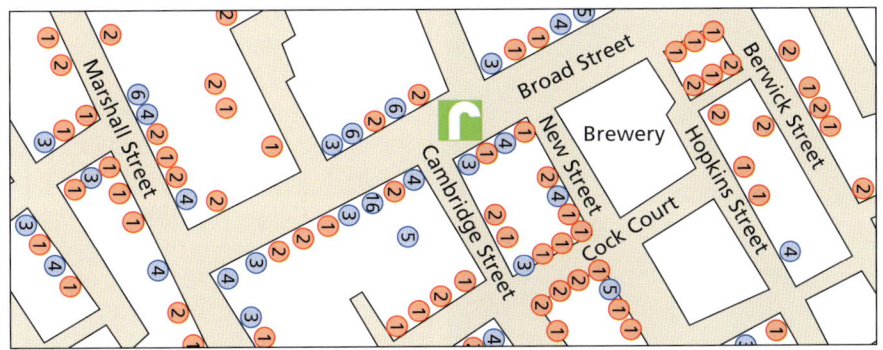

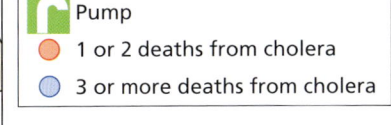

▲ **SOURCE P** A copy of part of Snow's map detailing deaths in the Broad Street area

The solution

Snow wrote a report on his findings. His evidence was so strong that the handle of the Broad Street water pump was taken away to stop people getting water from it. There were no more deaths. It was later discovered that a cesspool, only a metre away from the pump, was leaking into the drinking water. A woman living in Broad Street whose baby had contracted cholera had dumped a nappy into the cesspool.

The impact

Snow had proved that clean water was essential for preventing the spread of cholera, but this did not convince the government to act.

Many scientists still clung to the 'bad air' theory. Snow proved the link between the water and cholera, but could not explain *why* there was this link. It was not until after Pasteur published his Germ Theory that anyone could begin to understand exactly why the water was causing cholera.

There was a further cholera epidemic in 1865 which killed 14,000 people. But even this did not force the government to act. There were three main reasons why a new law was not passed:

- Wealthy people did not want to pay taxes to cover the cost of clean water supplies and sewers, which would benefit other people in the poor parts of their towns.
- Local councils did not want the national government interfering in how they ran their own towns.
- There was a strong belief in **laissez-faire** (governments should not interfere in people's lives) and self-help (people should help themselves to live better lives). Governments were still not expected to play a major part in improving the living and working conditions of the people.

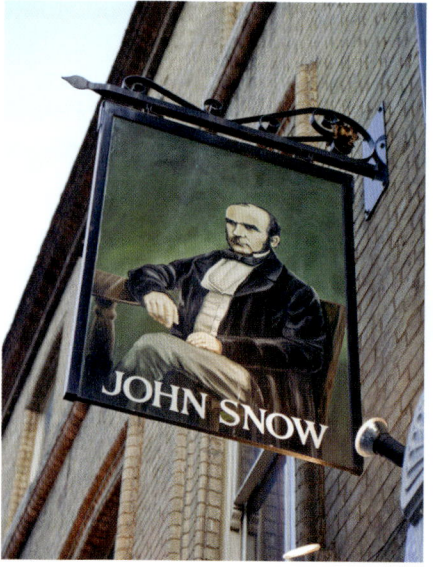

▲ This pub near the Broad Street pump was named in honour of John Snow

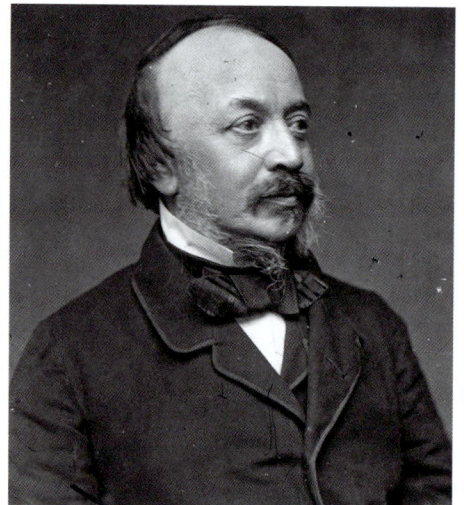

▲ Edwin Chadwick (1800-90)

What is public health?

Public health is organised by the government. Systems, such as fresh water, sewers and hospitals, are provided to the whole population to help prevent diseases spreading and in order that people become healthier. The government also makes laws to force towns and people to prevent diseases from spreading.

New approaches to prevention: The role of government and the Public Health Act (1875)

> **Research & Record**
>
> **Explain why there were improvements in public health in the nineteenth century.**
>
> Copy and complete the table below using the information on this page and on pages 74–75.
>
> Think carefully about the language you use to state how important each reason was. In column 2, choose a word or phrase from the scale on the right to show the level of importance. Do not fill in column 3 if you think a reason had no or only minimal impact.
>
> | Essential | No change could have happened without it |
> |---|---|
> | Important | Without it, change might have been less widespread or significant |
> | Minimal | Had only a little impact |
> | No importance | No influence at all |
>
> | Reasons for improvement in public health in the nineteenth century | Importance | Explanation |
> |---|---|---|
> | | | |
> | | | |

Edwin Chadwick

In 1842, a civil servant called Edwin Chadwick published 'A Report on the Sanitary Conditions of the Labouring Population'. Chadwick concluded that more people were dying from the unhealthy living conditions than died each year in wars. He said effective drainage and sewerage (sewer pipes to carry away waste) and clean water were needed. Chadwick was not the only person concerned about public health. In fact, much of the information came from interviews with and reports from local public health officers and doctors, especially in the big cities, but Chadwick was important in pulling the information together in a report and making sure that the government could not ignore what was happening.

The Public Health Act, 1848

In 1848, the government passed the first Public Health Act:

- A National Board of Health was set up.
- The government could force the local council to improve public health in towns where the death rate was high. This included improving the water supply and collecting sewage.
- Local councils were encouraged to collect taxes to pay for these improvements. However, this required support from local taxpayers.
- Councils were allowed to appoint medical officers of health to oversee public health.

The government had taken action by passing this Act, but towns did not have to carry out the improvements. They could improve public health if they wanted to and had support from taxpayers. This was a problem because nobody wanted to have their taxes increased! Some towns, including Birmingham and Liverpool, did make huge improvements. However, by 1853 only 103 towns had set up their own Boards of Health.

The lack of interest from town councils proved to be deadly. In 1854, Dr John Snow showed that cholera was caused by polluted water (see pages 74–76). In 1858, the River Thames was so polluted that it became known as the year of the Great Stink. Gradually, the pressure grew on the government and on local councils to act.

The Public Health Act, 1875

Finally, in 1875 a Public Health Act was passed that forced towns to make public health improvements. It was now compulsory for all local towns to improve sewers and drainage, provide fresh water and appoint medical officers and sanitary inspectors to check public health facilities.

Additional laws were passed that improved the standards of housing and stopped the polluting of rivers. This was important because most people got their water from rivers.

This Public Health Act was passed due to two developments in the nineteenth century:

- Louis Pasteur had proved that there was a scientific link between dirt and disease. Dr John Snow was able to prove that dirty water was the cause of cholera, even if he was not aware that it was bacteria in the water that was spreading this disease. When people had the scientific proof that clean water was needed, they were willing to pay higher taxes to cover the cost of public health improvements. With more support, towns began to make the changes needed.
- More working men in towns were able to vote for the first time in 1867. The number of working men voting increased again in 1884 when this right was extended to working men in the country. Politicians now had to improve the lives of working-class families to win the votes of working men. Many new laws were passed in the late nineteenth century to improve the lives of ordinary people in order to secure the votes of working men.

The reasons behind improvements in public health in the nineteenth century

1842 Chadwick's report (see page 77) highlights the link between illness and poor living conditions.

1854 Dr John Snow links cholera to infected water (see pages 74–76). His work showed the importance of using data to study epidemics. It also added to the pressure for clean water and effective sewerage systems.

1848 First Public Health Act (see page 77) allows, but does not force, councils to make improvements.

1858 'The Great Stink' (see page 77) added to the evidence that London needed a sewer system.

Summarise

The **SEWAGE** memory aid summarises Public Health changes in the nineteenth century.

Sewers open
Epidemics (for example, cholera)
Water unclean
Acts by government (for example, 1848 and 1875)
Germ Theory and Great Stink trigger action
Engineers improve sanitation (for example, Bazalgette)

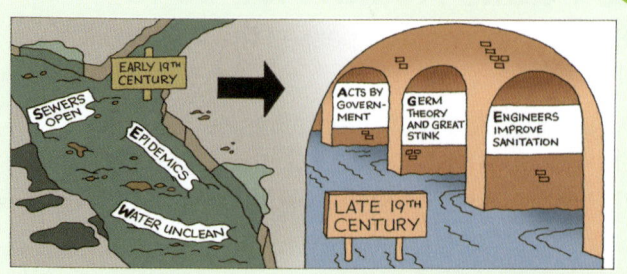

1860s Joseph Bazalgette organises the building of London's sewer system

In the 1850s, many people still believed that bad air (miasma) carried disease, so Londoners were scared by the Great Stink. This chance event forced MPs to take action to clean up the River Thames. They approved money to pay for a new sewage system for London.

It was a major engineering achievement which is still in use today. All London's sewage was pumped out of the city through:

- 83 miles of large sewers, built underground from brick
- 1100 miles of smaller connecting sewers from each street
- pumping stations at regular points to pump the sewage along the pipes.

This project was led by **Joseph Bazalgette**. During the Industrial Revolution, there had been great improvements in technology and engineering. Bazalgette used what he had learned in railway building to design and manage this project.

Most of the work was complete by 1865 and it led to significant improvements in the public health of London. But there was no public health act to enforce improvements throughout the country.

1875 A new and more effective Public Health Act

The 1875 Public Health Act finally **forced** local councils to improve public health. After this turning point, it was compulsory for local councils in each city or town to:

- improve sewers and drainage
- provide fresh water supplies
- appoint medical officers and sanitary inspectors to inspect public health facilities.

1900 Impact of medical developments

- Government intervention in the health of the people increased.
- More people had access to clean water.
- More vaccines were developed to prevent disease and illness.
- There were no more huge epidemics of cholera.
- Life expectancy increased.

1860s Pasteur's Germ Theory

Pasteur proved that there was a link between dirt and disease. The theory that illness was caused by 'bad air' finally faded away. This was a turning point. Faced with scientific proof, people were more willing to pay taxes to cover the costs of cleaning up their towns and cities, and more councils accepted responsibility to improve public health.

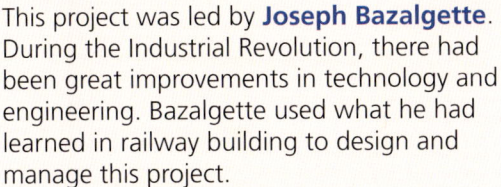

1867 More working men in urban areas get the vote

The number of voters increased. Now, if politicians wanted to win elections, they had to promise to do things to help working men, not just the wealthy and middle classes. The 1870s and 1880s saw many new laws passed designed to improve the lives of ordinary people.

1875–1900 More laws to improve public health

Laws were passed to:

- stop the pollution of rivers (from which people got water)
- shorten working hours in factories for women and children
- make it illegal to put unhealthy additives in food
- make education compulsory.

Part 3 Eighteenth- and nineteenth-century medicine period review

Review

What led to improvements in medicine during the eighteenth and nineteenth centuries?

Fill in a table like the one below to review the period. Use the cards at the bottom of the page to guide you.

Period summary, c1700 – c1900: Medicine in eighteenth- and nineteenth-century Britain			
Theme	**Improvements in the eighteenth and nineteenth centuries**	**Key individuals**	**Other factors**
Ideas about the cause of disease and illness	Reached a turning point: • From 1860s, the Germ Theory replaced bad air as an explanation for disease. • Microbes that cause individual diseases were identified.		
Approaches to prevention	Significant improvements in the nineteenth century: • Smallpox vaccination was made compulsory. • Other vaccinations were developed (e.g. anthrax, rabies). • Improvements were made in public health, including understanding the cause of cholera and increased government action. The Public Health Act of 1875 was a turning point.		
Approaches to treatment	More continuity than change: • Everyday treatments remained the same. Patent medicines were often worthless. • Improvements were made in hospital care and design. • Professional training of nurses was introduced following the work of Nightingale. • Improvements in surgery were made in dealing with pain (anaesthetics, e.g. ether and chloroform) and infection (antiseptics, e.g. carbolic acid and aseptic surgery).		

Individuals
- Edward Jenner
- Louis Pasteur
- Robert Koch
- Florence Nightingale
- James Simpson
- Joseph Lister
- Edwin Chadwick
- John Snow
- Joseph Bazalgette

Science and technology
- Better microscopes
- Improvements in chemistry
- Improvements in engineering

Government
- Political change (vote given to working-class men)
- Public Health Act of 1848
- Public Health Act of 1875

Attitudes in society
- Observation and experimentation
- Reduction in laissez-faire

Apply ▶ Recall Challenges

1 Sequencing

Sort these ten events from all three periods so far into chronological order:

Germ Theory	The Black Death
Smallpox vaccine	Thomas Sydenham and improved diagnosis
Discovery of the circulation of the blood	Discovery of chloroform
The Public Health Acts	Great Plague in London
The Royal Society	Discovery of the cause of cholera

2 Know the key individuals

Look at these key individuals:

- Louis Pasteur
- Robert Koch
- Edward Jenner
- Dr John Snow
- Florence Nightingale

For each one, try to answer these questions from memory:

- What contribution did they make to developments in medicine?
- What impact did they have?

Apply ▶ Exam Practice

Question 5/6 style

'The work of Edward Jenner was the most important development in medicine in the years c1700 to c1900.'
How far do you agree? Explain your answer.

(16 marks)

You may use the following in your answer:

- Smallpox vaccine
- Germ Theory

You **must** also use information of your own.

Exam Tip

Making a judgement (Question 5/6)

Look again at the advice on how to approach this type of question on page 29.

Remember to use the **3Ds**:

- **Decode** the question (work out the focus of the question).
- **Decide** how to organise your answer into paragraphs.
- **Develop** your answer by explaining and supporting the points you make. Explain why you agree and disagree that the work of Edward Jenner was the most important development in medicine. Support each argument with specific knowledge. Make sure you have included three aspects of knowledge across your whole answer.

In the exam, you must make a judgement about how far you agree with the statement. The easiest way to do this is to write a conclusion at the end of your answer. The best answers will have their overall judgement running throughout the answer. For example, when answering this question:

- Decide whether you agree or disagree that the work of Edward Jenner was the most important development in medicine. You could then begin your paragraph with: 'In conclusion, the work of Edward Jenner was the most important development in medicine because …'
- Go on to explain why you have reached this judgement by explaining the importance of the work of Edward Jenner. Consider the long-term impact or how many people he helped.

Part 4 Case study: Fleming, Florey and Chain's development of penicillin

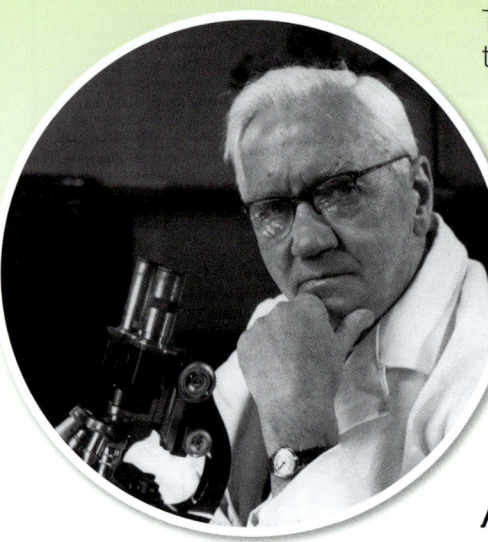

Connect & Engage – Alexander Fleming

This is **Alexander Fleming**. He played a significant role in one of the most important medical breakthroughs – the first antibiotic. An antibiotic is a drug made from bacteria that kills other bacteria and so cures an infection or illness.

War wounds

During the First World War, Fleming was sent to France to study soldiers' wounds. He found that wounds infected with bacteria were not healed by chemical antiseptics. Many soldiers were dying from their infected wounds.

Back home, Fleming worked on finding a way to deal with these bacteria. Ten years later, in 1928, Fleming found what he had been seeking.

A chance discovery

Fleming was working at St Mary's Hospital, London. When he went on holiday, he left a pile of petri dishes containing bacteria on his laboratory bench. On his return, he sorted out the dishes and noticed mould on one of them. Around the mould, the bacteria had disappeared.

He looked closer through his microscope and could see that the areas where the bacteria had died were covered with a mould called penicillin. He did not know where it had come from – it must have blown in through the laboratory windows that were open while he was on holiday.

Fleming then carried out experiments with the penicillin mould.

- He discovered that if it was diluted, it killed bacteria without harming living cells.
- He made a list of the germs it killed.
- He used penicillin successfully to treat another scientist's eye infection.

However, it did not seem to work on deeper infections and it was taking ages to create enough penicillin to use in his experiments, so he stopped his research.

Communicating his findings

Fleming did write up his experiments, however, and in 1929, he published his research in a medical journal, but nobody thought his article was important. Fleming discussed penicillin's potential as an antiseptic, but he made no great claims for its role as a general antibiotic. Fleming had not used penicillin to heal major illnesses, nor done systematic tests on animals. It went largely unnoticed … for now!

On pages 84–85 you will see what happened next.

Connect & Engage

How important was the work of Alexander Fleming?

Using these two pages:

1. Explain why Alexander Fleming's work was so important in the treatment of disease. Why was it a turning point? Think about how disease had been treated up until the 1920s.
2. Fleming may have discovered the properties of penicillin, but it needed other factors to turn his discovery into a life-saving drug. How many other factors can you identify? Make a list – you will need it for the task on page 84.

How has the treatment of disease developed since 1860?

Louis Pasteur
Pasteur publishes his Germ Theory in 1861. Doctors and scientists can now see the link between germs (microbes) and disease.

Robert Koch
Koch and his research team identify the specific microbes that were causing individual diseases. His methods also help others to do their own microbe hunting.

Joseph Lister
In 1872, Lister notices that the mould of bacteria called penicillin killed other bacteria. Years later, in 1884, he uses this mould to treat a nurse who has an infected wound. But Lister does not use it again. A miracle cure lies waiting for someone else to rediscover it.

Vaccinations
Scientists use Pasteur and Koch's work to develop a range of vaccinations.

Chemical cures
Scientists find **magic bullets** (chemicals) that kill particular infections inside the body.

In 1909, Paul Ehrlich develops Salvarsan 606, which destroys the bacteria that cause syphilis.

In the 1930s, Gerhard Domagk develops Prontisil, which kills the bacteria that cause blood poisoning.

Sulphonamide drugs
The chemical in both Salvarsan 606 and Prontisil is sulphonamide.

Drug companies start to mass-produce sulphonamide-based cures for diseases such as pneumonia and scarlet fever.

However, these magic bullets cannot kill **staphylococcus** germs, which cause major infections and often kill their victims.

Alexander Fleming

Key ideas or discoveries
In 1928, Alexander Fleming discovers that penicillin kills bacteria.

He publishes his findings in 1929 but his ideas are not taken up straight away by other scientists.

Short-term impact – the first effective antibiotic
In the 1930s, Howard Florey and Ernst Chain develop Fleming's idea into a medical treatment.

Penicillin becomes the first antibiotic.

Penicillin is used in the Second World War to treat Allied soldiers.

Long-term impact – antibiotics for all
Penicillin and other antibiotics are mass-produced by the **pharmaceutical industry**. In Britain, after the Second World War, the government provides antibiotics free to anyone who needs them through the National Health Service.

The impact of antibiotics in modern medicine has been far-reaching. It is no exaggeration to say that they have saved millions of lives.

Case study: Fleming, Florey and Chain's development of penicillin

Florey and Chain develop penicillin

Research & Record

How did factors affect the development of penicillin?

1. On page 82, you listed factors that were important in the development of penicillin. Use that list and these two pages to complete the explanation sentences in a copy of this table.
2. Use the Exam Tip on page 85 to write some explanation paragraphs.

Factor	Explanation – why was this factor important?
Individuals	Fleming deserves credit for the initial discovery. Florey and Chain were important because …
Government	The British government provided the funds for … The American government provided the funds for …
Science and technology	Without the pharmaceutical industry, it would not have been possible to …

Florey and Chain

In 1938, Howard Florey and Ernst Chain were working together at Oxford University, researching how germs could be killed. They read Fleming's article on penicillin and realised that it could be very effective, so they tried to get funding from the British government to manufacture penicillin. They only got £25! Still, Florey and Chain persevered.

They tested penicillin on mice and discovered that it helped mice recover from infections. However, to treat one person they needed 3000 times as much penicillin as they had used to treat one mouse. So they began growing penicillin wherever they could, using hundreds of hospital bedpans, even though the metal was in demand for building Spitfire aeroplanes.

By 1941, Florey and Chain had enough penicillin to test it on one person. Their volunteer was Albert Alexander, a policeman. He had developed septicaemia (blood poisoning) from a tiny cut. The penicillin worked and Alexander began to recover. However, the penicillin ran out after five days. Florey and Chain were so desperate to continue the treatment that they extracted unused penicillin from the man's urine and reused it. Eventually, the penicillin ran out and the policeman became ill again and died. However, Florey and Chain had proved that penicillin worked and that it wasn't harmful to the patient. Their big question now was how to make enough of it.

Mass production

English factories were too busy making war supplies to help, so Florey went to the USA – at just the right time. In 1941, the USA was attacked by the Japanese at Pearl Harbour and entered the war. The US government realised the potential of penicillin for treating wounded soldiers and made interest-free loans to US companies to buy the expensive equipment needed for making penicillin. By 1944, there was enough to treat all the Allied wounded on D-Day in June – over 2.3 million doses.

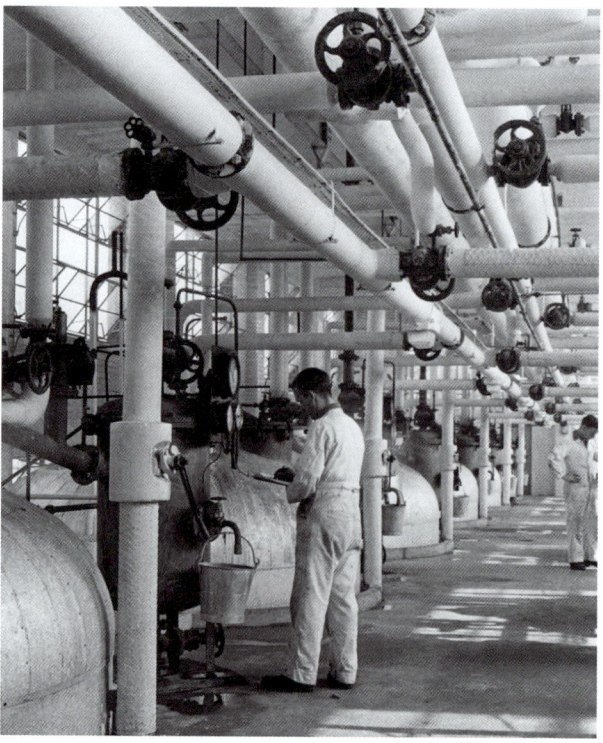

▲ **SOURCE A** Tanks used to produce penicillin

Antibiotics for everyone

War led to the development of penicillin. It led to government investment and proved that penicillin could transform the treatment of many illnesses.

However, once the war ended in 1945, there was still a lot to do to make antibiotics available for the whole population.

- Pharmaceutical companies paid for researchers to discover and trial other antibiotics.
- Scientific techniques and technological equipment were improved to enable this work.
- After 1948, the government-funded NHS provided antibiotics free of charge.
- Scientists and doctors communicated their research so they could learn from each other.

The development of antibiotics transformed medicine. Before antibiotics, pneumonia, meningitis and similar infections often killed their victims. Afterwards, people were much more likely to survive.

Fleming's discovery set off a chain of events that saved millions of lives.

Apply ▶ Exam Practice

Question 4 style

Explain why medical treatment improved in the modern period. (12 marks)

You may use the following in your answer:
- Development of penicillin
- Lung cancer

You **must** also use information of your own.

Exam Tip

Support your answer with specific knowledge

The first sentence makes the argument clear – a reason for improved treatment in the modern period.

Possible answer

Medical treatment improved in the modern period because of the investment and support from government. In 1938 the British government invested £25 into Florey and Chain's research of penicillin. This enabled Florey and Chain to test penicillin on mice and prove that it helped them to recover from infections. However, during the Second World War ...

Precise knowledge is being used to support the argument and prove the reason is correct.

This paragraph should be completed with more supporting knowledge which should be linked back to the question.

Summarise

Here is a visual summary of the penicillin story. Penicillin made Fleming **FAMOUS**.

Fleming ... discovers first ...
Antibiotic ... made from ...
Mould ... developed into penicillin by ...
Others ... Florey and Chain who travelled to the ....
USA ... to raise funds for use on ...
Soldiers ... in the Second World War.

Turn this into your own memory aid by adding your own pictures for each stage. Keep it simple – do not spend a long time on your drawings. The important thing is that they are memorable to you, not that they are brilliant artwork.

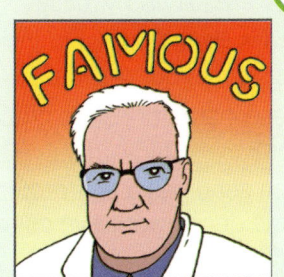

Part 4 Ideas about the cause of disease and illness c1900–present

Advances in understanding the cause of illness and disease: The influence of genetic factors

Research & Record

How has the understanding of genetic illnesses developed in modern Britain?

Pasteur's discovery of Germ Theory was a huge advance in medicine. It led to many changes in preventing and treating illness. However, there were still illnesses that could not be explained by germs. Understanding of genetic disease and illness developed in the second half of the twentieth century after DNA was discovered in 1953.

Use the information on pages 86–87 to complete your own copy of this bingo card.

Discovery of DNA bingo		
What is **DNA**?	What are **genes**?	**When** was DNA discovered?
Give two advances in technology that enabled the discovery of DNA.	What were Crick and Watson able to **prove about DNA**?	**How** did the British government help the discovery of DNA?
How did the mapping of a human genome advance understanding of medicine?	**Name three** genetic illnesses.	**How** has knowledge of genes developed our understanding of breast cancer?

The influence of genetics: The discovery of DNA

DNA

DNA (deoxyribonucleic acid) is in every cell of our bodies.

The structure of DNA is a pair of interlocking spirals. We call this a double helix.

They are joined by 'bases', set in pairs.

DNA is like a long list of instructions that operates each cell in our bodies.

These instructions are grouped together. We call them **genes**.

Each gene has a different function, for example some decide your eye colour or your hair colour, and some decide whether you will have a disease or a disability.

Everybody has different DNA with different instructions. This is what makes us all different.

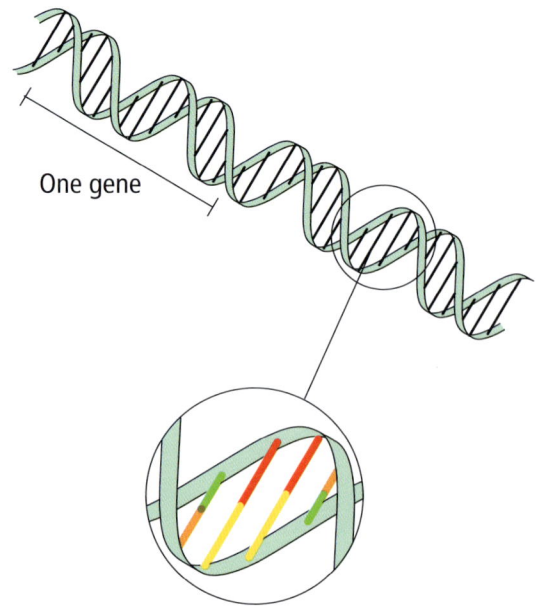

▲ **SOURCE B** A section of DNA

The discovery of DNA took place over a series of discoveries.

The first discovery took place in 1953 when Francis Crick and James Watson, two scientists in Cambridge, discovered the structure of DNA (see Source B). They were able to make this discovery because of advances in technology. The electron microscope allowed scientists to see smaller objects in much finer detail. **X-rays** had also improved. X-ray photographs could now be taken using a technique called crystallography, which uses **radiation** to take the high-power photograph. Using these developments, Crick and Watson were able to prove that DNA was in every human cell and passed information on from parents to children. Crick and Watson were helped by a team of scientists with different skills. Maurice Wilkins was an expert in X-ray photography. Rosalind Franklin had developed a technique to photograph a single strand of DNA. She was the first person to take X-ray photographs of DNA. Working as a team, they carried out experiments that other scientists had not tried. Their experiments cost a great deal of money. Most of this money was given to them by the government and industry.

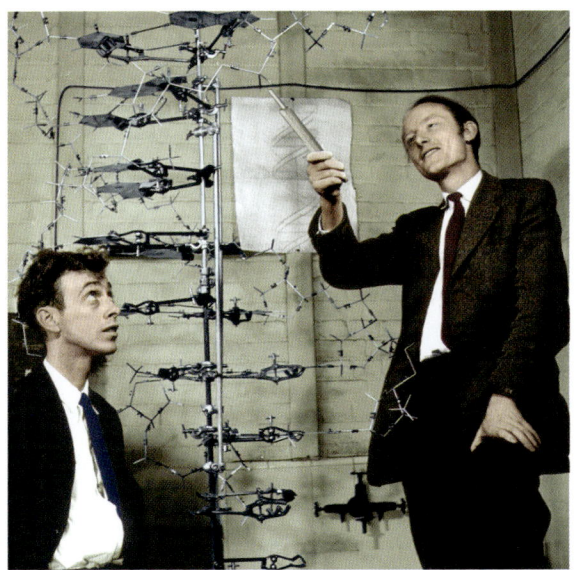

▲ **SOURCE C** Francis Crick and James Watson with a model of the structure of DNA

Mapping the human genome

In 1986, the Human Genome Project began. Its aim was to identify the exact purpose of each gene in the human body to compile a complete map of human DNA. This project took years and was completed in 2001. A complete set of genes in a living creature is called a genome.

A team of scientists in 18 countries, including the United States, Britain and Japan, were involved in the research for this project. Computers were an essential part of their work, and the research could not have taken place without them. Information was stored and shared using computers and the internet. The information carried in human DNA would fill 80,000 books.

Once the human genome had been mapped, it was possible for scientists to look for mismatches in the DNA of people suffering with hereditary diseases.

Why is DNA so important to the history of medicine?

Many illnesses have genetic causes. They are inherited in the genes of the person who has the illness. Scientists have discovered that there are specific genes that pass on conditions and illnesses such as diabetes, cystic fibrosis, Down syndrome and some forms of cancer.

It is hoped that scientists can find ways to help those who have these illnesses.

Knowledge about genes has been used to develop our understanding of breast cancer. Scientists have now been able to identify a gene that can be present in women who have this illness. This knowledge cannot be used to treat breast cancer. However, women who have this gene identified can undergo a range of treatments to prevent breast cancer. In the most severe cases, they might require a mastectomy, an operation to remove their breast.

Advances in understanding the cause of illness and disease: The influence of lifestyle factors

Research & Record

How has understanding of the impact of lifestyle factors on our health developed in modern Britain?

Use pages 88–89 to complete your own copy of a table like this. Record examples of the ways in which our lifestyle can affect our health and examples of diseases and illnesses linked to lifestyle factors.

Ways in which our lifestyle can affect our health	Examples of diseases and illnesses linked to lifestyle factors

The influence of lifestyle factors on health

The twentieth century has also seen a development in knowledge about and understanding of the effect that our lifestyle can have on our health. In previous centuries, the major killers tended to be the result of environmental factors, diseases spread by close contact or underlying poor health of victims. In the modern period, Britain began to become more prosperous. Most people were wealthier, better fed, had more leisure time and worked less and, as a result, they lived longer. However, these improvements in lifestyle have resulted in new health problems.

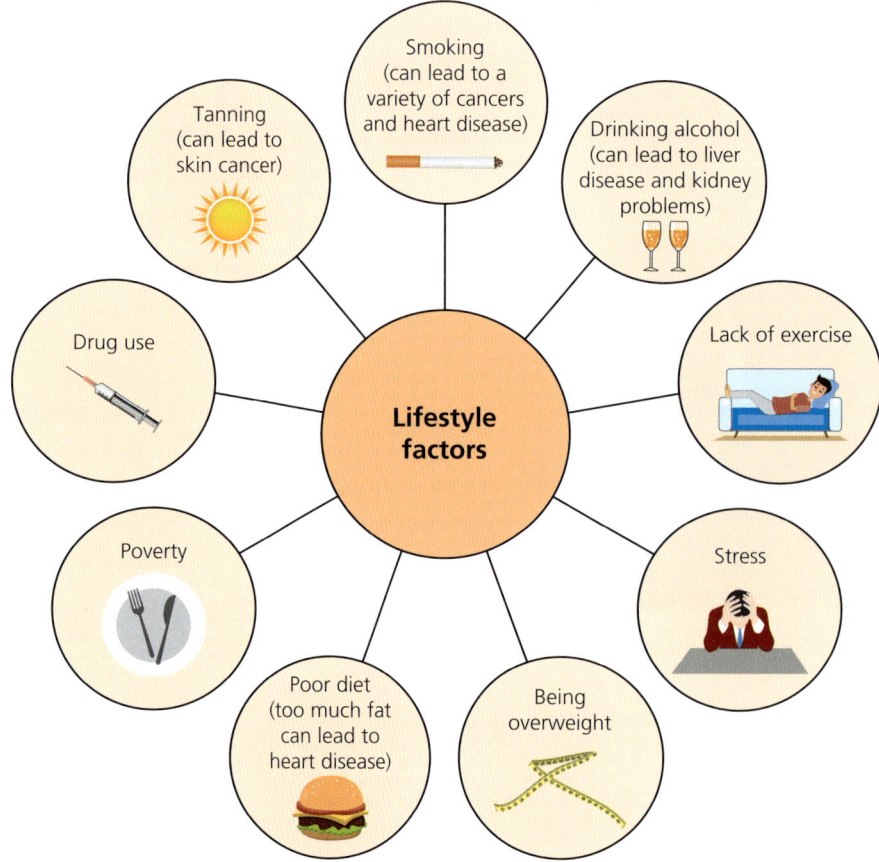

▲ Lifestyle factors that can cause health problems

Today, the big killers are heart diseases, respiratory diseases, liver disease and dementia. We also seem to have greater mental health problems like depression, although it may be that we are now simply more aware of mental health problems. All these major lifestyle factors can lead to disease and illness, such as a variety of forms of cancer, heart disease, type 2 diabetes, asthma and mental health problems. Research is taking place all the time, paid for by the government, universities and some medical organisations. Smoking is the biggest cause of preventable diseases in the world.

Linking a healthy lifestyle to preventing illness was not a new approach. Hippocrates recommended diet and exercise to avoid poor health and this advice continued in medieval England. However, what was new after c1900 was that features of people's lifestyle choices could be linked more closely to specific diseases. For example, we now know that a poor diet can lead to heart diseases.

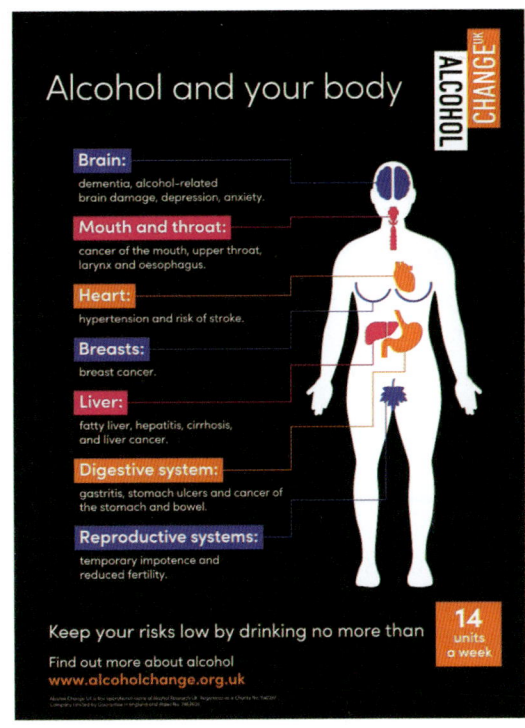

▲ **SOURCE D** A poster from the charity Alcohol Change UK, showing the diseases and health issues linked to drinking alcohol

Apply ▶ Exam Practice

Question 3 style

Use the Exam Tip below to help you answer this question:

Explain **one** way in which understanding of the cause of disease and illness in the nineteenth century was different to understanding of the cause of disease and illness in the twentieth century. (4 marks)

Exam Tip

Comparing time periods (Question 3)

Look again at the advice on how to approach this type of question on page 39.

Remember to focus on explaining a difference and supporting your explanation with an example from both time periods.

- Think about the developments in the understanding of the cause of disease and illness.
- Think about who made the discoveries that developed this understanding.

Improvements in diagnosis

Research & Record

How has the diagnosis of disease and illness advanced since c1900?

Read pages 90–91.

1. Create a mind map detailing the ways in which disease and illness have been diagnosed since c1900.

2. Use this information and the factors in the table below to write two paragraphs explaining why there have been advances in the diagnosis of disease and illness since c1900. You will not use all of the factors below. Choose two that enabled advances in the diagnosis of disease and illness.

| Individuals | Government | Church | Science and technology | Attitudes in society |

Diagnosis is the process that takes place to identify the disease or illness someone is suffering from. Improvements in science and technology have led to advances in diagnosis in the twentieth and twenty-first centuries.

Technology

Developments in technology have led to machinery being created that can diagnose an illness exactly. These machines cost a lot of money and have been funded by the government, medical companies and universities. Some machinery can be purchased and used at home, such as machines that monitor blood pressure and blood sugar levels, as well as heart monitors and cholesterol monitors.

Science

Alongside improved technology, scientific knowledge and understanding of the human body has increased. This has enabled medical professionals to examine human body cells to diagnose disease and illness.

Attitudes

Developments in scientific understanding of the human body alongside advances in technology have led to people trusting medical procedures and being willing to go for scans and tests to diagnose disease and illness. These advances have increased the trust that society has in science and medicine to diagnose and explain disease and illness.

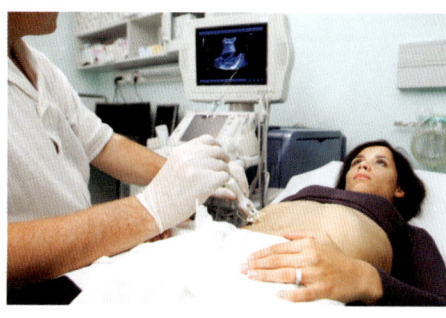

▲ **SOURCE E** A doctor performing a liver biopsy and using an ultrasound

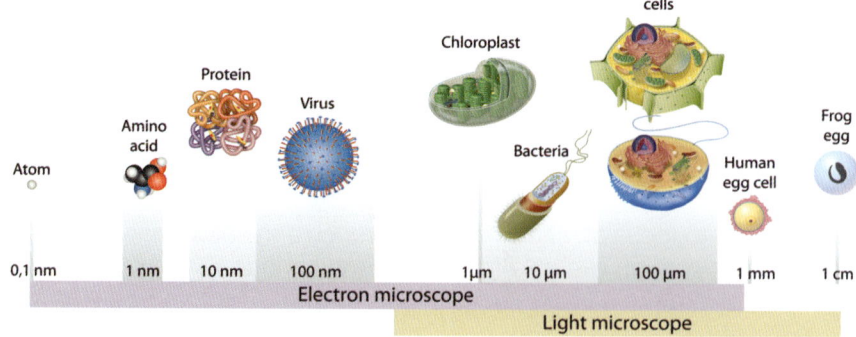

▲ **SOURCE F** A diagram showing the increased power of electron microscopes over normal microscopes

Blood tests
Blood samples are used to test for medical conditions.

Blood sugar monitoring
People who suffer from diabetes are able to test their blood sugar regularly so that they can manage their illness.

Electron microscopes
This is a very strong microscope that allows doctors to see very small objects such as human cells.

Blood pressure monitors
These are used to diagnose high and low blood pressure.

X-rays
These allow a doctor to see inside the human body without using surgery. They are used to identify broken bones.

MRI scans
These create an internal image of the body using magnets and radio waves. They are used to identify soft tissue injuries such as ligament damage.

ECGs (electrocardiogram)
These are electrical impulses used to monitor heart activity.

Endoscopes
An **endoscope** is a camera on the end of a thin, flexible wire. It is used to see inside the human body without using surgery. It is often used to investigate digestive symptoms, such as vomiting blood.

Nuclear medicine
Radioactive elements are injected into a patient's bloodstream. This allows a doctor to track and diagnose changes in the body through disease.

CT scans
These are a more advanced form of X-ray and are used to identify growths in the body such as tumours.

Ultrasound scans
These create a picture of the inside of the body using sound waves. They are used to diagnose kidney stones and gall stones.

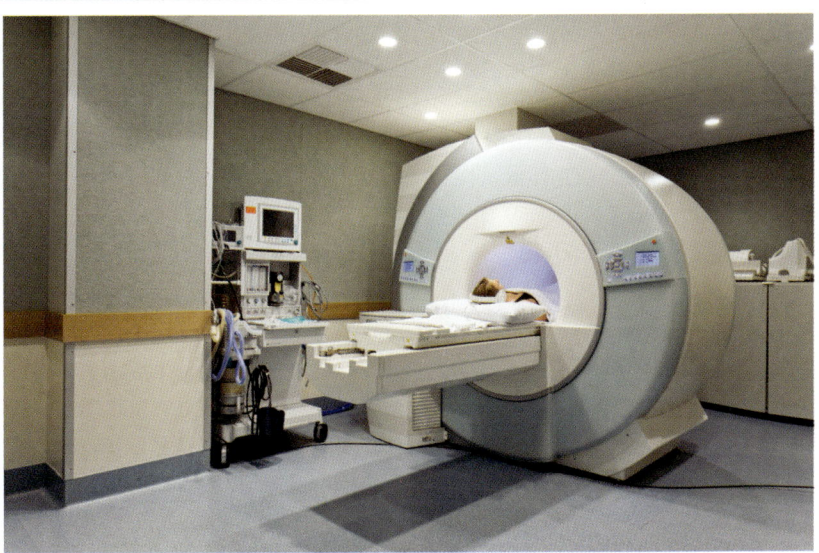

▲ **SOURCE G** A CT scanner

Improvements in diagnosis

Part 4 Approaches to prevention and treatment c1900–present

Improved access to care: Government reform

Research & Record

Who benefitted from government reforms in the early twentieth century?
Use pages 92–93 to complete your own copy of this bingo card.

Government reforms bingo		
What percentage of recruits were rejected during the Boer War because they were unfit?	**At what age** could people get an Old Age Pension after 1908?	**Which group** of people benefitted from the National Insurance Act after 1911?
Give two ways that Booth and Rowntree influenced the actions of the Liberal Government.	**How** did health visitors support mothers after giving birth?	**Which two groups** paid into the National Insurance scheme, apart from workers?
What was the infant mortality rate in 1900?	**Give three examples** of how schoolchildren benefitted from Liberal social reforms.	**List three groups** of people who did not benefit from the National Insurance Act.

Demands for reform

By 1900, life expectancy was starting to rise. It had reached 46 for men and 50 for women. Towns were cleaner. Public health facilities were beginning to improve. But the key words here are 'starting to' and 'beginning to'.

The problem of poverty

Many people still suffered major health problems, partly because of dirt but even more because of poverty. The government gave no help to the sick, unemployed or elderly. Those who could not get help from friends and relatives or charities had to go into a workhouse, run by the local council. The infant death rate (see Source H) was still very high. One in seven babies died before they reached their first birthday.

Researchers such as Charles Booth and Seebohm Rowntree published reports that showed just how poor many people were and also showed the links between poverty and ill health.

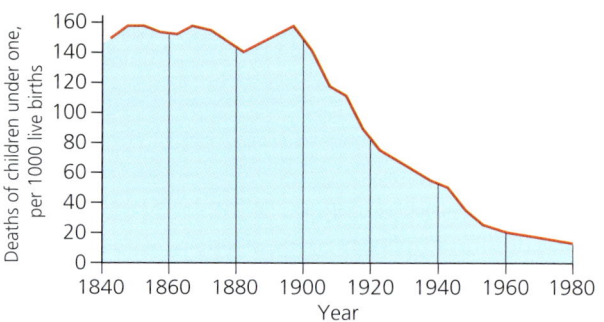

▲ **SOURCE H** The death rate of children under one year old, 1840–1980. Infant mortality rates have fallen dramatically since the early twentieth century

Possibly even more shocking to the government was the finding from medical inspections when they tried to raise an army to fight the Boer War that began in 1899. An incredible 38 per cent of all potential recruits were unfit to serve on medical grounds. Governments might not have thought solving the problem of poverty was their job – but having a strong army was!

Government reforms in the early twentieth century

In 1906, a new Liberal Government was elected by a vast majority. Their election campaign had included promises to tackle poverty – and they delivered on this promise. From 1908, David Lloyd George served as Chancellor of the Exchequer and introduced a series of radical reforms to finance and taxation. These reforms may seem ordinary today, but a hundred years ago they were revolutionary.

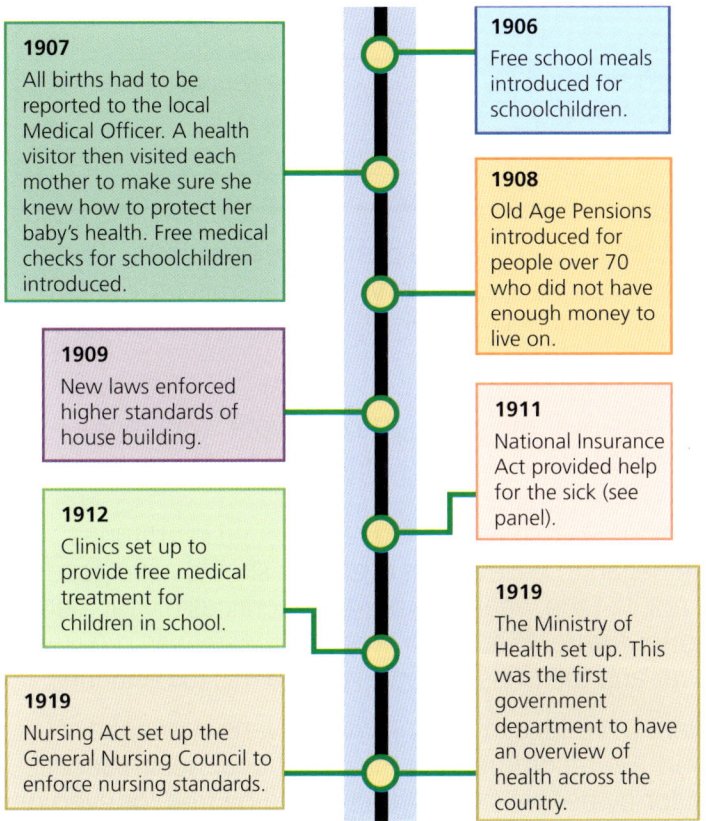

1906 Free school meals introduced for schoolchildren.

1907 All births had to be reported to the local Medical Officer. A health visitor then visited each mother to make sure she knew how to protect her baby's health. Free medical checks for schoolchildren introduced.

1908 Old Age Pensions introduced for people over 70 who did not have enough money to live on.

1909 New laws enforced higher standards of house building.

1911 National Insurance Act provided help for the sick (see panel).

1912 Clinics set up to provide free medical treatment for children in school.

1919 The Ministry of Health set up. This was the first government department to have an overview of health across the country.

1919 Nursing Act set up the General Nursing Council to enforce nursing standards.

National Insurance Act, 1911

This was one of the greatest changes introduced by the Liberal Government. It gave workers medical help and sick pay if they could not work through illness. Until then, workers who fell ill had a choice: carry on working although they were ill, or not work and get no pay, which usually meant they could not afford medical help either.

The **National Insurance** scheme required the worker, his employer and the government to pay into a sickness fund. (The government contributed 2d per week, the employer 3d and the worker 4d.) When a worker fell ill and was unable to work, he received 10d a week for up to 26 weeks and free medical care. This was paid out of the sickness fund. It was a major step forward, although it only covered people in work, not their families. Most women and all children were excluded. So were the unemployed, the elderly and anyone who had a long-lasting illness.

Summarise

The Liberal reforms … **OPENS** the door for further public health improvements:

Old Age
Pensions
Education for mothers
National Insurance
School meals and medical checks

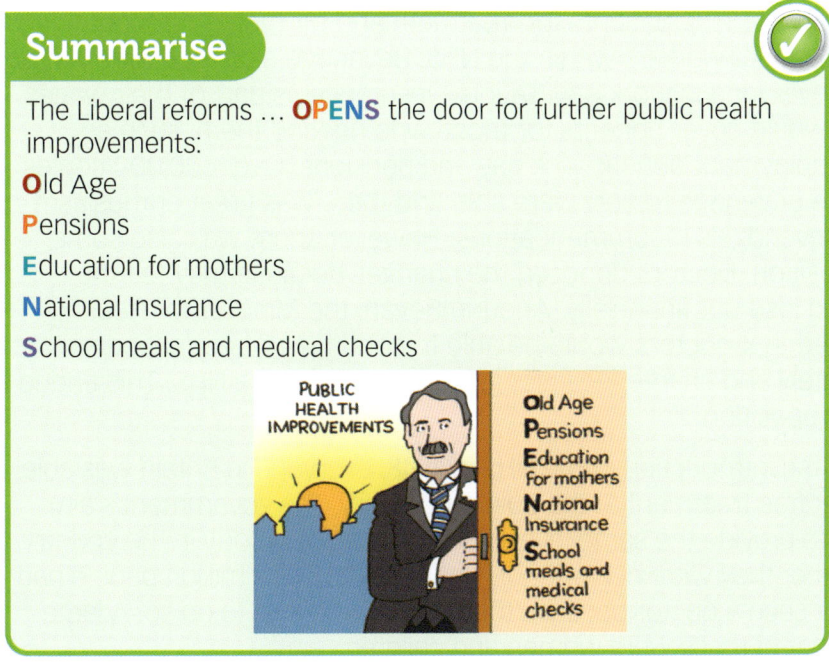

Improved access to care: Impact of the NHS

Research & Record

Why has access to care improved in the years since c1900?

Complete the table below using the information on pages 92–95. You will be able to use these notes to answer the exam question on page 105.

Argument	Supporting evidence
Access to care has improved since c1900 because of more intervention from government.	Evidence of more intervention from government:
Access to care has improved since c1900 because attitudes in society have changed.	Evidence of a change in attitudes in society:

The greatest change in medical care came in 1948 with the introduction of the National Health Service (NHS). This provided free healthcare at the point of delivery for all.

Why was the NHS introduced?

- By 1928, all adults over the age of 21 could vote. With more working people able to vote, the government had to make changes to improve healthcare.
- The Second World War (1939–45) led to a change in attitudes. More people began to believe that everyone should have good healthcare, not just the wealthy. After the sacrifices of war, people wanted a better future. In addition, free healthcare was provided during the war and the British people wanted this to continue.

In 1942 Sir William Beveridge, a leading civil servant, wrote the Beveridge Report. He recommended that a National Health Service be set up, paid for by people's taxes, that would be free for everyone to use. He wanted doctors, nurses and other medical workers to stop charging patients for treatment and for them to become government workers within the NHS. Beveridge also recommended that everyone in work pay National Insurance as part of their wages. This would cover benefits for those who needed them, such as unemployment benefit, sick pay and pensions. Over 600,000 copies of the Beveridge Report were sold and there was great enthusiasm for Beveridge's recommendations. However, there was also some opposition. Doctors opposed the changes because they felt they would lose out financially. Aneurin Bevan, the Minister for Health, agreed that doctors would be able to continue to treat patients privately and charge fees alongside working for the NHS. This ended the opposition.

With the introduction of the NHS in 1948, everyone in Britain was able to get free treatment at the point of delivery. The government's aim was to provide the same level of service for everybody in the country, whether they were rich or poor. Until 1948, about 8 million people had never seen a doctor because they could not afford to do so. A large number of these were women and children.

The diagram below shows the range of services available:

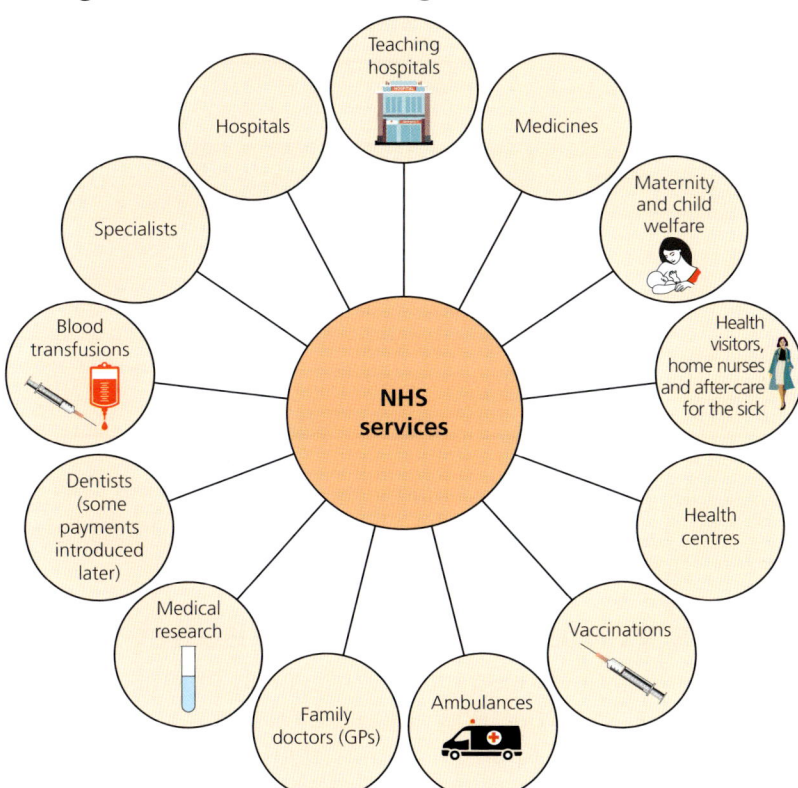

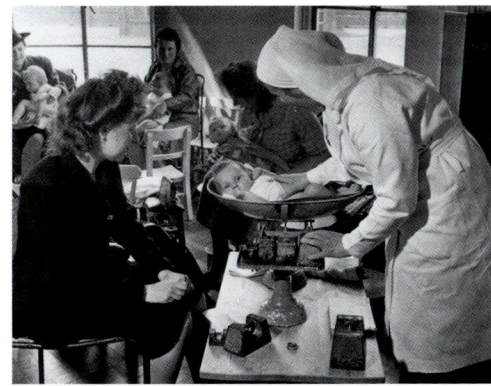

▲ **SOURCE I** A Bristol clinic, 1948. This was one of the free services provided by the newly established NHS

In addition to the above, new equipment was provided. After initially relying on previous hospital buildings, new hospitals were built from the 1960s. Since 1948, the government has spent money on improving specialist care in hospitals. Nurses and doctors can now develop in specialisms such as **paediatrics**, emergency medicine or supporting cancer patients undergoing radiotherapy or **chemotherapy**.

Hospitals today also have to protect patients from acquiring new illnesses and infections while in hospital, such as **MRSA**. The Care Quality Commission has been set up to check care in hospitals and to insist on improvements if needed.

Summarise

1. Can you remember why the changes introduced by the Liberal Government between 1906 and 1919 were important? Use the **OPENS** memory aid to help you.
2. Complete the memory aid below. Explain each of the phrases alongside the NHS ambulance. Why was the introduction of the NHS so significant?

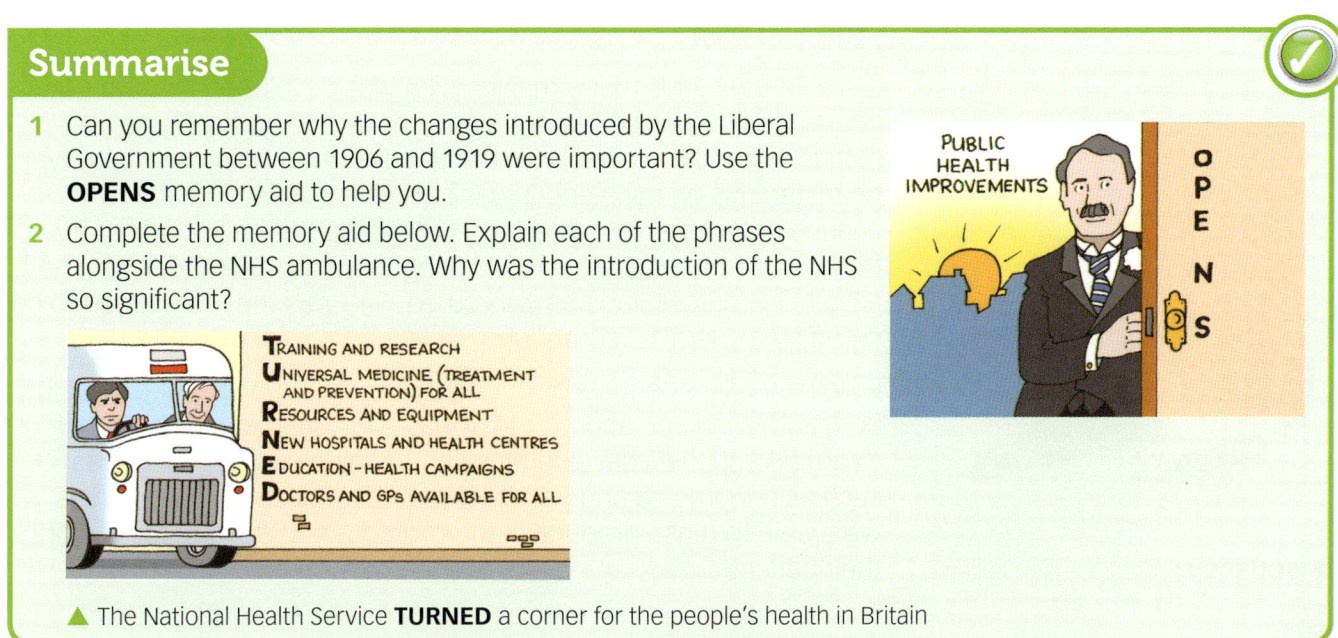

▲ The National Health Service **TURNED** a corner for the people's health in Britain

The impact of science and technology

Research & Record

What impact did science and technology have on medicine after c1900?

Use pages 96–97 to complete your own copy of a table like this. Record example(s) of developments in medical treatment and surgery due to advances in science and technology.

Developments in medical treatment	Developments in surgery

As well as leading to changes in diagnosis, science and technology have also led to great changes in the way disease and illness have been treated since 1900.

Advances in medicines: Magic bullets

In 1909, Paul Ehrlich developed the first 'magic bullet'. This was a chemical drug that killed bacteria inside the human body. Ehrlich was a member of Robert Koch's research team in Germany. He used the work of Koch to identify microbes and applied it to a treatment for disease and illness. It was called a magic bullet because when the chemical entered the body it attacked a specific microbe and killed it.

The first magic bullet was Salvarsan 606 and it destroyed the bacteria that caused syphilis. Syphilis had been a disease that many suffered from throughout the eighteenth and nineteenth centuries. Ehrlich tested a number of arsenic **compounds** to find a cure. The 606th compound that he tested was successful in attacking the microbe. He was helped by a Japanese scientist called Sahachiro Hata.

It was in the 1930s that a magic bullet was developed that did not contain arsenic and therefore kill the patient. Gerhard Domagk tested a chemical called Prontosil to cure blood poisoning. Initially, he tested this on mice and it was successful. He then had the chance to test it on a human when his daughter became very ill from a cut from a rose bush. His daughter would have died, but he gave her Prontosil and she was cured. She was the first human to be cured by a chemical compound.

Following this, scientists discovered that the important chemical in both Salvarsan 606 and Prontosil was sulphonamide. This led to drug companies developing sulphonamide cures for diseases such as pneumonia and scarlet fever. Pharmaceutical companies were able to mass-produce it and promote it to doctors for use on their patients.

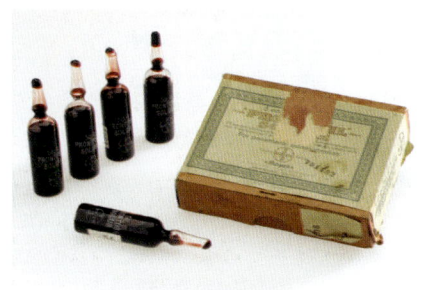

▲ **SOURCE J** Prontosil, magic bullets

Antibiotics

Earlier in this book we covered the story of penicillin. Penicillin was the first antibiotic, a drug made from bacteria that killed other bacteria to cure an infection or illness. You can remind yourself using pages 84–85.

Following the discovery and development of penicillin during the Second World War, the government did a great deal to make it available for the whole population. Money was invested into the discovery and development of other antibiotics by pharmaceutical companies. Technology was developed to mass-produce antibiotics. After 1948, the NHS provided antibiotics for free until prescription charges were introduced in 1952. Today, many different antibiotics are used including penicillin, tetracycline and gentamicin.

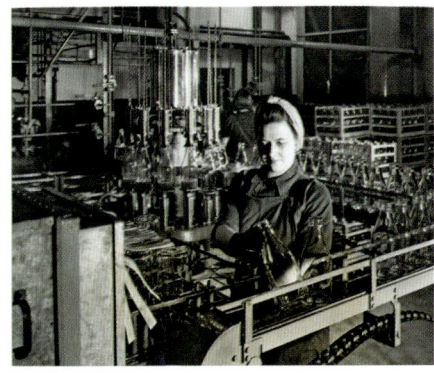

▲ A penicillin production line, 1944

Apply ▶ Exam Practice

Question 3 style

Explain **one** way in which the treatment of disease and illness in the years c1250 to c1500 was different from the treatment of disease and illness in the years c1900 to the present.   (4 marks)

Exam Tip

Comparing time periods (Question 3)

Look again at the advice on how to approach this type of question on page 39.

Remember to focus on explaining a difference and supporting your explanation with an example from both time periods.

- Think about the approaches to treatment during the Black Death in 1348.
- Compare this with the chemical cures that have been used to treat disease and illness since c1900.

Research & Record

How important was science and technology for advances in medicine after c1900?

Use pages 98–99 to complete the table you started on page 96.

Think carefully about the words you use to evaluate the importance of science and technology. How was each development essential to medical progress?

Essential	No change could have happened without it
Important	Without it, change might have been less widespread or significant
Minimal	Had only a little impact
No importance	No influence at all

High-tech medical and surgical treatment in hospitals

Hospital treatments have changed a lot since 1900. Due to advances in science and technology, treatments take place today that would not have existed before 1900.

Prior to c1900, blood loss had been a major cause of death in surgery. In 1909, Karl Landsteiner discovered three blood groups – A, B and O – and soon a fourth was discovered, AB. This scientific knowledge solved the problems faced when attempting **blood transfusions** from one person to another. The discovery of blood groups enabled blood transfusions to take place after blood types had been matched. With the problem of blood loss solved, more complex operations could take place.

1 Radiation therapy and chemotherapy

Radiation therapy (or radiotherapy as it is also called) developed from Röntgen's discovery of X-rays.

Marie Curie, a Polish scientist, played a very important role. While she was researching X-rays with her husband, Pierre, they noticed that the skin on their hands was burned by the material they were handling. This led to the discovery of radium, which has been used ever since to diagnose and to treat cancers. Sadly, Marie Curie herself died of leukaemia, caused by the radioactive material she used in her research.

Radiotherapy aims to kill the cancer cells using beams of radiation. Techniques have improved to target cancers more precisely.

Since the 1970s, chemotherapy has been used if the cancer has developed so far that surgery and radiotherapy are not successful. Chemotherapy involves using particularly powerful chemicals to attack the cancer cells, although it can have significant side effects because healthy cells are killed too.

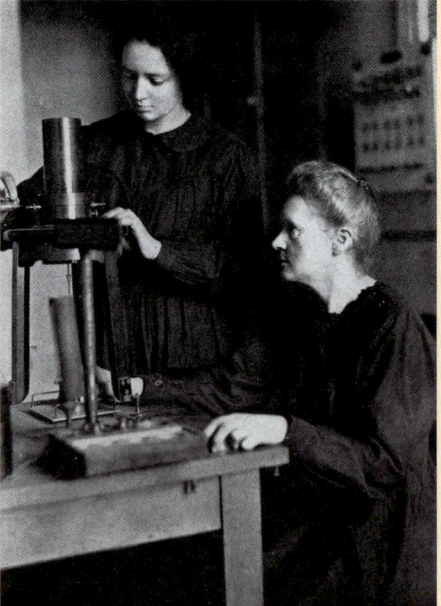

▲ **SOURCE K** Marie Curie (1867–1934), with her daughter in 1920. She is the only woman to have won two Nobel Prizes, for her work on X-rays and on radium

2 Plastic surgery

Plastic surgery and skin grafting techniques continued to develop after the First World War (see page 128). These have had a huge impact on modern surgery and have helped individuals to overcome the emotional and psychological effects of severe injuries.

3 Open-heart surgery

Improvements in technology have led to dramatic advances in heart surgery. The heart/lung machine was designed to bypass the heart and maintain blood circulation while surgery is carried out on the stopped heart. This enabled surgeons to replace diseased valves or repair defects in the walls between the chambers of the heart. By the 1970s, heart bypasses had become common and heart surgery quite routine.

4 Transplant surgery

The first heart **transplant** was carried out in South Africa in 1967. Other organs had been transplanted before then (kidneys in 1954 and a liver in 1963) and, since then, even more ambitious transplants have been carried out, including the first bone marrow transplant in 1980, the first heart and lung transplant in 1982, and the first womb transplant in 2023.

All transplants depend on technical skill and many other discoveries. For example, before transplants could work, scientists had to discover drugs to stop the patient's body rejecting their new replacement organs.

5 Keyhole surgery

Major surgery used to mean surgeons making large cuts into the body. Nowadays, large incisions are avoided as often as possible. Instead, **keyhole surgery** allows surgeons to work through a tiny hole to carry out complex operations.

This is possible because of miniaturisation – all the surgeon's tools are inside a small instrument called an endoscope which is controlled by the surgeon using miniature cameras, fibre-optic cables and computers.

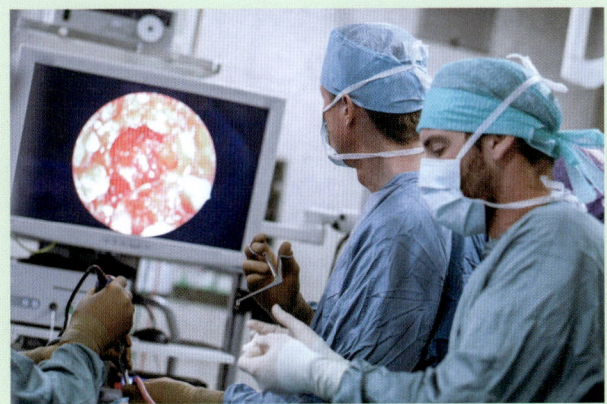

▲ **SOURCE L** Keyhole surgery being used to carry out a procedure

6 Robotic surgery

Surgeons can now use robots to carry out some operations. Robots can be more precise and controlled than human surgeons. Nanobots (tiny specialised robots less than a millimetre long) can perform tasks such as clearing arteries.

Apply ▶ Exam Practice

Question 4 style

Explain why developments in science and technology led to rapid progress in medicine in the years c1900–present. (12 marks)

You may use the following in your answer:
- Magic bullets
- Chemotherapy

You **must** also use information of your own.

New approaches to prevention

Research & Record

How far did approaches to the prevention of disease and illness change after c1900?

1 As you read through pages 100–101, use a table like this to record the continuity and change in approaches to the prevention of disease and illness after c1900.

2 Then evaluate how much change this period saw in approaches to the prevention of disease and illness. Choose the appropriate phrase from the scale below and explain why you have come to this conclusion.

Evidence of continuity in approaches to the prevention of disease and illness after c1900	Evidence of change in approaches to the prevention of disease and illness after c1900

A total change in …   Significant change   Some changes but mainly continuity   Considerable continuity   No change in …

3 Choose the strongest piece of evidence to support your overall conclusion.

Mass vaccinations

After the positive impact of the smallpox vaccination programme (see page 71), other government vaccination programmes followed in the twentieth and twenty-first centuries to tackle the most serious diseases. However, vaccine is no longer compulsory but encouraged by the government.

As a result of the vaccine and widespread advertising campaign, measles is now very rare, although it is not completely wiped out. Influenza is another disease that can lead to death, especially in elderly people. As a result, governments have invested money in providing free vaccines for vulnerable groups of people.

Vaccination programmes
- 1896 Typhoid
- 1906 Tuberculosis (TB)
- 1913 Diphtheria
- 1927 Tetanus
- 1952 Whooping cough
- 1954 Polio
- 1964 Measles
- 1988 MMR (measles, mumps, rubella)
- 2008 Human papillomavirus (HPV)
- 2015 Meningitis B
- 2020 Covid-19

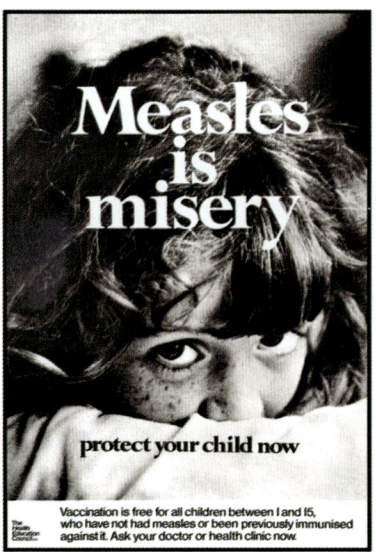

▲ **Source M** A government advertising campaign for the measles vaccine in the 1950s

Government lifestyle campaigns

The role of government in medicine has changed through the twentieth century and into the twenty-first century. The government now takes action to educate people so that they can prevent disease and illness. The government does this by using various different strategies:

- Advertising campaigns to warn against the dangers to health, such as smoking, recreational drug use and binge drinking.
- Initiatives that encourage people to eat more healthily and do more exercise, such as the Change4Life campaign.
- Events that encourage people to adopt a healthier lifestyle, such as Stoptober which encourages people to stop smoking and Dry January which encourages people to avoid drinking alcohol for a month.
- Health checks offered every five years to everyone over the age of 40, which look at blood pressure, weight and cholesterol levels.

Coronavirus disease, 2019

The Coronavirus disease 2019 is also known as Covid-19. The first known case was identified in December 2019 and quickly spread worldwide, leading to the Covid-19 pandemic. Symptoms of Covid-19 include fever, cough, headache, fatigue, breathing difficulties, loss of smell and loss of taste. Most people who catch the virus develop mild symptoms. Older people are at a higher risk of developing severe symptoms. Some people are affected by the virus for years after infection. This is called Long Covid. Many studies are taking place across the world to investigate and understand the longer-term effects of the disease.

During the Covid-19 pandemic, the British government tried to prevent the spread of the disease using a combination of legislation, education and campaigns. The government introduced legislation that enforced physical or social distancing, quarantining and the use of face masks in public. They also educated people on how to reduce the chance of catching Covid by improving the ventilation of indoor spaces and careful handwashing. A vaccine was developed in 2020 to try to prevent the spread of the virus.

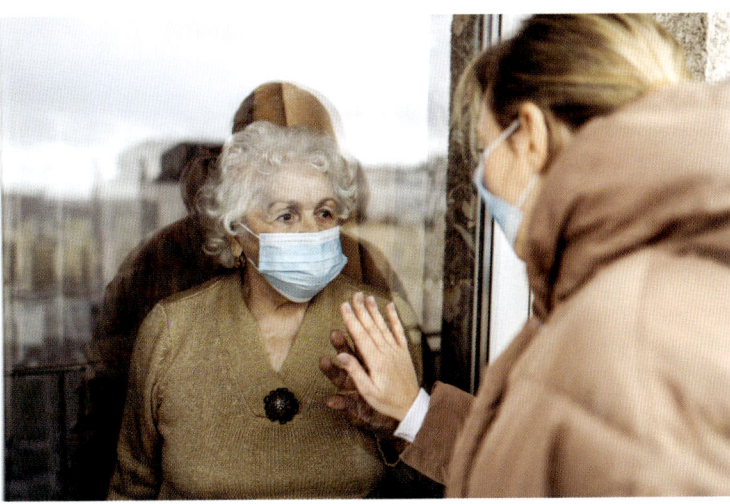

◀ A woman looking through a window at a family member who is in quarantine

Part 4 Case study: The fight against lung cancer in the twenty-first century

Research & Record

Explain why there has been progress in the fight against lung cancer in the twenty-first century.

Read pages 102–103. Copy and complete the table to record your findings. Aim to identify at least two main reasons.

Identify a reason	Support with examples	Explain why this has led to progress in the fight against lung cancer

Today, lung cancer is one of the most common forms of cancer. In the UK, over 40,000 people are diagnosed with it each year. The seriousness of lung cancer has meant that great efforts are being made to improve its prevention, diagnosis and treatment.

Cause

Medical evidence has proven that cigarette smoking is the major cause of lung cancer. Nearly 90 per cent of cases are the result of smoking, and this includes passive smoking (breathing in other people's tobacco smoke).

Prevention

Many people die from lung cancer because it is so difficult to diagnose in its early stages. It is diagnosed once the symptoms are evident and so, by this time, the cancer may have spread. Only a third of lung cancer patients live for as long as a year after diagnosis. Only 10 per cent live for longer than five years. There is a much lower survival rate for lung cancer patients compared to patients of other cancers.

The government has made a huge effort to try to prevent lung cancer using the following methods:

- Major advertising campaigns have been used to emphasise the dangers of smoking and campaigns have educated people about the symptoms to encourage early diagnosis.
- Advertisements for cigarettes have been banned.
- Shops can no longer have cigarettes on display.
- Laws have been passed that make it illegal to smoke in public places, such as cafes, restaurants and workplaces.
- In 2007, the legal age for buying tobacco was raised from 16 to 18 years.
- Taxation on tobacco products has been increased.

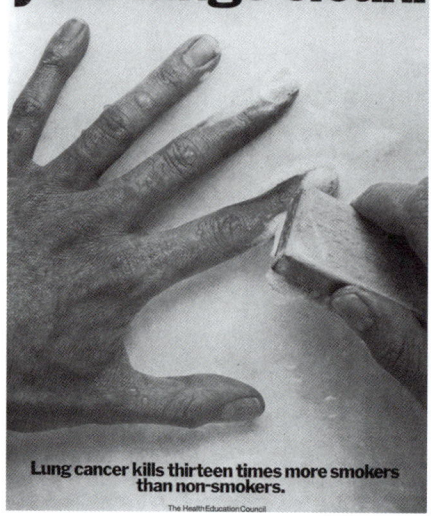

▲ SOURCE N An NHS anti-smoking poster from the 1980s

The use of science and technology in diagnosis and treatment

Governments have also invested large amounts of money in improved treatments. This has been implemented through the NHS. Scientists have taken part in research programs to learn more about the disease and money has been invested in new technology. The screening of high-risk individuals is being developed, but there is currently no national screening programme because the technology needed to detect the earliest signs of lung cancer has not yet been developed. A CT scan (see page 91) is used to detect cancer in a patient's lungs before a bronchoscope is used to collect some of the patient's lung cells.

Treatments for lung cancer include:

- **Surgery**. An operation can take place to remove the tumour, a small piece of the patient's lung or the entire lung. However, this has proven dangerous because lung cancer patients also suffer from other smoking-related illnesses. New surgery techniques using remote-controlled micro-instruments and cameras have far less impact on the body and allow for a speedy recovery.
- **Radiotherapy**. Radiation beams are used to shrink and kill the cancer cells and radiotherapy is used to prevent tumours from growing bigger. Techniques have been developed that target the cells more precisely.
- **Chemotherapy**. Powerful chemical medicines are used to attack the cancer cells. This form of treatment is only used if surgery and radiotherapy have been unsuccessful because a patient can experience serious side effects. New forms of chemotherapy are constantly being trialled by scientists trying to find a more effective treatment.
- **Immunotherapy**. Trials have been taking place to boost the immune system and help it to block the growth of cancer cells and tumours.

The fight against lung cancer in the twenty-first century shows how a number of factors now work together for progress in medicine. Here we can see the government working alongside science and technology to tackle one of the biggest killers in our society.

Apply ▶ Exam Practice

Question 3 style

Explain **one** way in which the role of government in medicine in the years c1700 to c1900 was similar to the role of government in medicine in the years c1900 to present. (4 marks)

Part 4 Medicine in modern Britain period review

Review

What led to improvements in medicine in modern Britain?

Fill in a table like the one below to review the period. Use the cards at the bottom of the page to guide you.

c1900–present: Medicine in modern Britain				
Theme	Improvements in modern Britain	Role of government	Science and technology	Other factors
Ideas about the cause of disease and illness	Developments in understanding since the middle of the twentieth century: • From the 1950s, understanding of genetic illness developed after the discovery of DNA. • More recently, there is an understanding that our lifestyle has an impact on our health. • There have been improvements in the diagnosis of disease and illness.			
Approaches to prevention	New approaches to prevention: • Mass vaccinations are available to prevent many diseases. • Government lifestyle campaigns educate us on how to prevent illness and disease.			
Approaches to treatment	Significant improvements since c1900: • Magic bullets and chemical cures have been developed. • Antibiotics have been developed after the initial discovery of penicillin. • Medical and surgical treatments available in hospitals have increased. • The NHS enables free access to care and treatment for all at the point of delivery.			

Individuals
- Paul Ehrlich
- Gerhard Domagk
- Alexander Fleming
- Howard Florey
- Ernst Chain
- Marie Curie
- Francis Crick and James Watson

Government
- 1911 National Insurance Act
- 1948 National Health Service
- Lifestyle campaigns

Science and technology
- Understanding of DNA
- Radiation and chemotherapy
- Developments in chemicals
- Antibiotics
- Developments in engineering

Attitudes in society
- A belief that everyone should be able to access the same healthcare (after Britain's experience in the Second World War)
- Understanding of the impact of our lifestyle on our health

Apply ▶ Exam Practice

Question 3 style

Explain **one** way in which ideas about prevention of illness in the nineteenth century were similar to ideas about the prevention of illness in the twentieth and twenty-first centuries.

Apply ▶ Exam Practice

Question 4 style

Explain why government action in medicine has changed in the years c1700 to present. **(12 marks)**

You may use the following in your answer:
- Public Health Act (1875)
- Lung cancer in the twenty-first century

You **must** also use information of your own.

Exam Tip

Explaining change or continuity (Question 4)

Look again at the advice on how to approach this type of question on page 45.

Remember to use the **3Ds**:

- **Decode** the question (work out the focus of the question).
- **Decide** how to organise your answer into paragraphs.
- **Develop** your answer by explaining and supporting the points you make. Explain why government action in medicine changed. Support each reason with specific knowledge. Make sure you have included three aspects of knowledge across your whole answer.

Apply ▶ Exam Practice

Question 5/6 style

'In the years c1800–present day, the work of John Snow was the most significant development in approaches to the prevention of disease and illness.'

How far do you agree? Explain your answer.

(16 marks)

You may use the following in your answer:
- Broad Street pump
- Vaccination

You **must** also use information of your own.

Exam Tip

Making a judgement (question 5/6)

Look again at the advice on how to approach this type of question on page 29.

Remember to use the **3Ds**:

- **Decode** the question (work out the focus of the question).
- **Decide** how to organise your answer into paragraphs.
- **Develop** your answer by explaining and supporting the points you make. Explain why you agree and disagree that the work of John Snow was the most significant development in approaches to the prevention of disease and illness. Support each argument with specific knowledge. Make sure you have included three aspects of knowledge across your whole answer.

When you decode the exam question, look carefully at the dates for the period that you need to focus on. Hopefully you have noticed that in the question above you are asked about the period c1800 to the present day. Some questions will ask you to consider medical developments across two chronological periods.

Part 5 How do we know about injuries and treatments in the British sector of the Western Front, 1914–18?

Research & Record

What sources do historians use to find out information about injuries and treatments during the First World War?

In this part of your course, you are going to study how medicine responded to the challenges of a particular historic environment – the British sector of the Western Front in the First World War. You will also be explaining how sources are useful for your study. You will also think about how you might further investigate particular aspects of the topics.

Use the examples on these two pages to gather examples of the sources that historians use. Present your examples as a mind map or list.

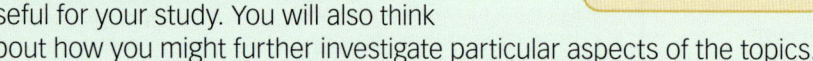

Medical sources for the First World War

Personal letters

You have probably been studying history for many years in your school career. You have probably used many history books in these lessons. You have probably also used sources and answered questions on them. You may not have thought too much about where the authors of the history books found the information they used to write their books. The short answer is that they use sources. 'Sources' is the term we use for anything that historians can gain information from. Historians use a great many written sources. These can be official documents, but they can also be personal letters, diaries, song lyrics, tax bills – almost anything. Historians sometimes use artefacts as well. These are objects that shed light on some aspect of the past.

What makes sources useful?

In your exam paper you will get a question about sources. You will be asked to study some and explain how useful they are.

Historians do this too. However, there is an important point to realise here. Historians do not ask *whether* a source is useful, they ask *how* it is useful. In other words, all sources are useful as evidence about something.

Historians make a source useful by using the content and provenance of the source alongside their own knowledge.

Content

Historians make a source useful by making observations and inferences from the information in the source. Observations are what we can read or see in the source – what it says. Inferences are where we find out something from the source that it may not tell us directly – what we can infer.

Provenance

Historians make a source useful by considering the type of source (nature), who the source came from and when (origin), and why the source was created (purpose).

Knowledge

Historians make a source useful by comparing the content of the source with their own knowledge and using their own knowledge to understand the importance of the provenance. For example, if a source was created in the summer of 1916 on the Western Front, they would know that this was at the time of the Battle of the Somme (see page 111).

What types of sources can be used?

In the reference section of her book *Medicine in the First World War Europe*, the historian Fiona Reid lists the different types of sources she used. Here are just a few:

- Personal letters, for example from ordinary soldiers, medical officers, family members
- Official letters by government officials, or military personnel
- Memoirs, diaries and personal stories
- Paintings and photographs
- Medical textbooks from 1914–18, particularly military medical textbooks
- Military training manuals
- Casualty records such as medical field cards
- Orders and bills for medicine, bandages and other medical equipment
- Articles in newspapers and magazines
- The publications of particular organisations like the British Medical Association
- Employment records and contracts showing wages, holidays, etc.

More recently, Lindsey Fitzharris has written a book about the First World War surgeon Sir Harold Gillies (see page 128). In the reference section of her book, *The Facemaker*, Fitzharris also lists the different types of sources she used. These include:

- Personal letters
- Newspaper articles
- Army reports
- Diary entries
- Photographs
- Articles in medical journals such as *The Lancet*

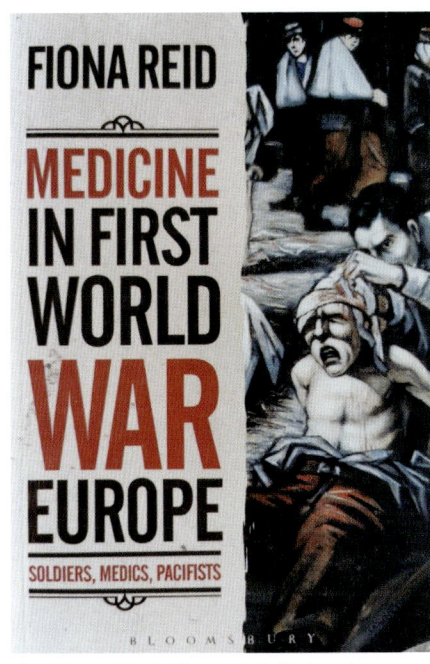

▲ **SOURCE A** Fiona Reid's book, *Medicine in the First World War Europe*

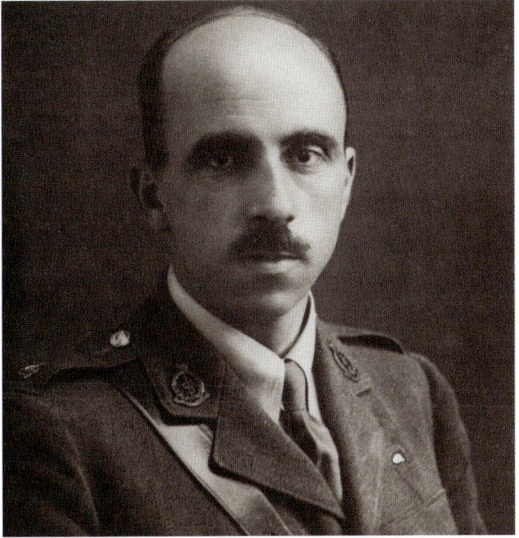

▲ Harold Gillies (1882–1960)

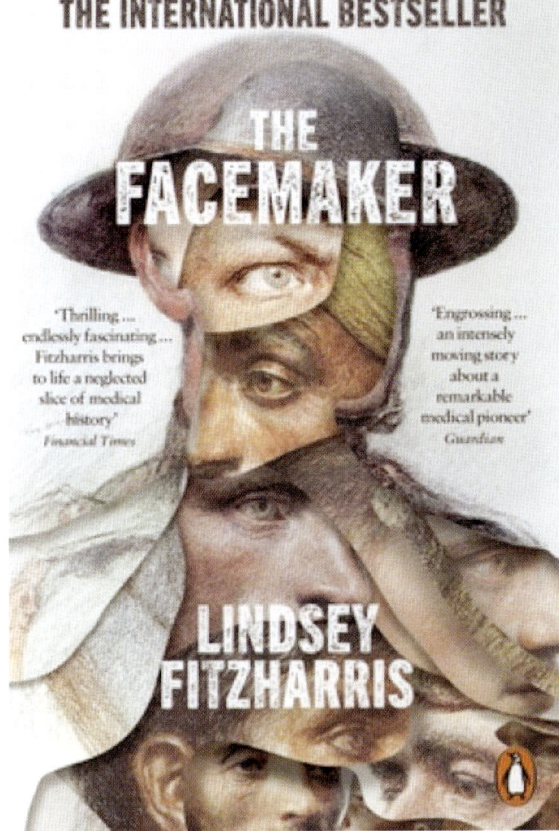

▲ **SOURCE B** Lindsey Fitzharris' book, *The Facemaker: One Surgeon's Battle to Mend the Disfigured Soldiers of World War I*

Part 5 The historical context of medicine in the early twentieth century

> ### Research & Record
>
> **How did medicine advance in the early twentieth century?**
>
> As you have seen from pages 54–79, medicine developed in major and important ways in the 1800s. Not surprisingly, this continued in the early 1900s as well. There were improvements in many areas. On these pages (108–109) we are going to look at three important areas which would eventually become important on the Western Front. Use a table like this to record details of the advances in medicine in the early twentieth century.
>
> | Advance | Details |
> |---|---|
> | Understanding of infection | |
> | Development of X-rays | |
> | Blood: transfusions and storage | |

Understanding of infection and developments in aseptic surgery

During the 1800s there were great advances in surgery. The introduction of anaesthetics transformed surgery. However, a continuing problem was that even after a successful operation, patients could pick up infections and often died. In the 1860s, the pioneering surgeon Joseph Lister, building on the work of scientists like Robert Koch and Louis Pasteur, introduced techniques for antiseptic surgery. This meant preventing patients being infected by using carbolic acid to sterilise the surgeon's scalpels and other instruments, and using **ligatures** (threads which sewed up wounds). Lister's results were very impressive.

Other surgeons built on Lister's ideas and by the 1890s hospitals were moving from antiseptic surgery (which killed germs in the operating theatre) towards aseptic surgery, where they tried to eliminate germs from the theatre altogether. Operating theatres were cleaned. Instruments were heated with steam to kill germs. Surgeons and other medical staff had to wash their hands thoroughly and wear sterilised gowns, gloves and face masks.

The development of X-rays

In 1895, the German researcher Wilhelm Conrad Röntgen was doing experiments with cathode ray tubes. These were glass tubes filled with gas. Röntgen wanted to see what happened when he put an electric current through the tube. He covered the tube in black paper but to his surprise he discovered that some rays passed through the paper and showed up on the wall. Röntgen had accidentally discovered X-rays. He and many others quickly realised how valuable this could be. In medicine, a broken leg or arm could be exposed to X-rays. The X-rays passed through the flesh of the limb but not the bone. The X-rays then made a mark on photographic film. X-rays became a sensation in the medical world and beyond.

The machinery for X-rays was large, expensive and easily broken. It took a long time to produce an image and some early pioneers and patients were badly affected by radiation poisoning. Despite this, the use of X-rays was a massive advance in diagnosing and treating injuries. Less than six months after the discovery, hospitals were using X-rays. In London, Glasgow and Birmingham, hospitals opened new radiology departments.

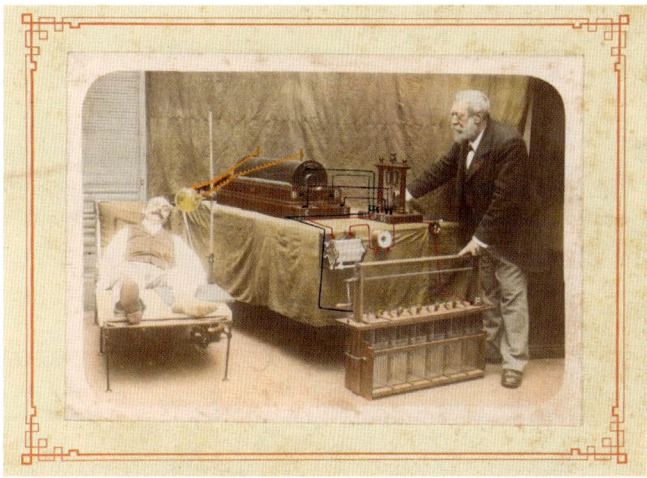

▲ **SOURCE C** A photograph from the Wellcome Collection showing a man having an X-ray on his leg in 1898

Blood: Transfusions and storage

As well as infection, another common problem with surgery around 1900 was loss of blood. Doctors had been trying to come up with a solution to the problem since the 1600s but attempts to give a patient more blood – known as blood transfusion – had never been successful.

The real breakthrough in this area came in 1901 when an Austrian doctor called Karl Landsteiner discovered that there were different blood groups and that a person with one blood type could not receive a different type of blood. Landsteiner discovered three blood groups – A, B and O – and soon a fourth was discovered, AB. Suddenly, it was possible to do blood transfusions safely and reliably as long as the donor and the patient had the same blood group.

There was one further problem, which was that blood could not be stored because soon after it left the human body it coagulated (thickened into **clots**). As long as the donor and the patient were close by *and* not too much blood was needed then this was not a problem.

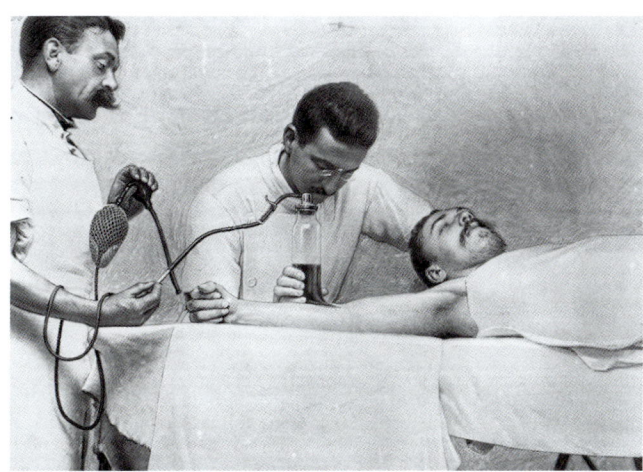

▲ **SOURCE D** A photograph of a blood transfusion from around 1900

The theatre of war in Flanders and northern France

Research & Record

What problems were experienced by those trying to help the wounded on the British sector of the Western Front?

Use pages 110–111 to complete your own copy of a table like this. Record details and possible problems for the four key areas of the British sector listed in the table. 'Terrain' means the physical features of a piece of land.

	Detail(s) of the terrain and/or key points of the battle(s)	Possible problems experienced by those trying to help the wounded
Ypres Salient and Hill 60		
Somme		
Arras		
Cambrai		

Tension had been building between the great powers of Europe in the early 1900s. In 1914, the tension exploded into war. Britain, France and Russia fought against Germany and Austria–Hungary. The war was fought in many different parts of the world, and by soldiers from many different countries (on these pages, 'British' forces could also include soldiers from the British Empire, including India, Australia, Canada, the Caribbean and many more). We are going to focus on the Western Front. The British sector of the Western Front was located in Flanders, a region in the north of Belgium, and northern France.

▲ **SOURCE E** The Western Front towards the end of 1914. The lines changed relatively little until early 1918

The Ypres Salient and Hill 60, 1914–17

Ypres was a beautiful medieval city. It was a key target for the Germans when they attacked in 1914 and it remained an important location throughout the war. If the Germans had captured Ypres, it would have opened the roads to the ports of the English Channel and could have cut off the supply lines for the British forces.

There was a bulge in the German lines around Ypres which was known as the Ypres Salient. This bulge protected the city but it meant that the city could be attacked from several directions. Because of its importance, there was almost continuous fighting around Ypres throughout the war, leaving the city in ruins.

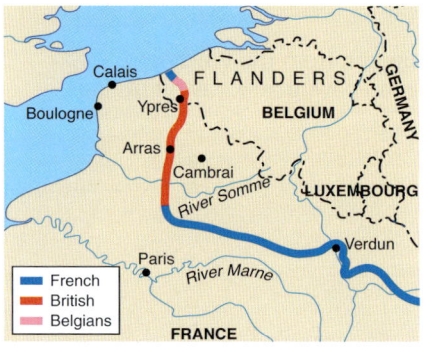

▲ **SOURCE F** The Ypres Salient, 1914–17

- In the First Battle of Ypres (October–November 1914), British, French and Belgian forces were able to halt the German advance, but the losses were heavy with around 95,000 casualties on all sides.
- In December 1914, the Germans captured important high ground surrounding Ypres, including the man-made hill called Hill 60. The British recaptured the Hill in April 1915 by planting and exploding mines underneath. The miners tunnelled under Hill 60 and planted five massive explosive mines. When they exploded them, the blast blew the top off the hill and enabled the British to capture it.
- Soon afterwards, the Germans attacked in the Second Battle of Ypres. The battle lasted one month. It was significant because it saw the first use of poisonous chlorine gas in war, causing massive casualties and a huge psychological shock. The British suffered around 59,000 casualties in the battle.
- In 1917, the British and their allies attacked the Germans in the Third Battle of Ypres. The battle lasted from 31 July to November 1917. The Germans were driven back but the British suffered around 245,000 casualties.

The Battle of the Somme, 1916

From February to July 1916 the Germans had been attacking the French at Verdun, causing massive losses. To relieve the pressure on Verdun, British and French forces attacked the Germans on 1 July 1916 at the Battle of the Somme. There were some important new tactics used during the battle. For example:

- The **creeping barrage** involved British artillery firing just ahead of the advancing troops in order to keep defenders pinned down in their trenches.
- Tanks were used for the first time in September 1916, but their impact was limited because of technical problems.

The battle achieved its aim of taking pressure off the French, but the costs were high. There were around 57,000 British casualties on the first day (about one in ten). The battle continued until November, with around 950,000 casualties on all sides.

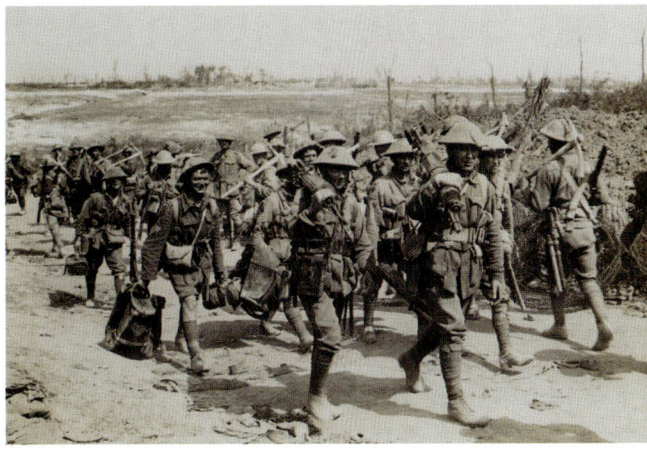

▲ **SOURCE G** A photograph from the National Army Museum showing British troops at the Battle of the Somme in the summer of 1916. A machine gun team is walking towards the camera while a trench digging team is walking away

The Battle of Arras, 1917

Arras saw plenty of fighting but probably the most significant event was in 1917. The land around Arras is mostly chalk and there were many natural caves. Tunnels were built and the caves were extended, using them as shelter for storing equipment, as a safe way to travel around and even as an underground hospital. In early 1917, they built up forces in these tunnels and launched a surprise attack on the Germans in April. The Battle of Arras brought a significant advance of around 8 miles, but the advance gradually slowed. Once again casualties were very heavy, at around 160,000.

Cambrai, 1917

Cambrai was held by the Germans for much of the war and was an important part of the German road and rail network for supplying troops. The British recognised its importance and launched a major attack in October 1917. The battle was significant because it was the first large-scale use of tanks, around 500 of them. The British also used a shorter artillery barrage which gave the Germans less warning of the attack. Once again, the British managed an initial advance but they found it hard to hold on to the land they had taken and eventually lost most of it.

Part 5 The British sector of the Western Front

Research & Record

What were the challenges of helping the wounded on the Western Front?

The fighting on the Western Front took place in the trenches. Use a table like this to record the challenges that the Western Front posed to those trying to help the wounded in the First World War. Note that you will need to add to your table after reading pages 112–114, so leave lots of space.

Feature	Challenge
Crooked trenches	Difficult to carry the wounded to a place for treatment

The trench system

The war began with massive German advances in the summer of 1914. British, French and Belgian forces just about managed to hold the Germans by autumn 1914. Each side was unable to defeat the other and so both sides began to dig trenches to protect themselves. From 1915 to early 1918, the trenches developed from simple shelters against enemy fire into sophisticated networks of trenches, tunnels, dugouts and bunkers. Soldiers advanced into battle from the frontline trenches. Behind these, support trenches were dug to hold extra troops and equipment. Source H shows what a section of the trenches looked like at the time.

Communications trench – supplies, ammunition and fresh troops came up these trenches.

Machine gun posts – they were deadly against attacking forces.

Dugouts – vital for protection against artillery. Artillery killed more soldiers than any other weapon. It could also cause psychological problems. This was usually called '**shell shock**'. Soldiers suffering from shell shock often became totally confused or lost their memories.

The trenches are crooked. This was a defensive measure. If a shell exploded in a trench, the blast would be contained. Also, if enemies captured one section, they could not shoot along the whole trench.

Support trench – extra troops would be based here in case there was an attack on the front line. There would be further **reserve trenches** behind the support trench.

Barbed wire – often 20–30 metres deep, impossible to get through unless you knew where the gaps were. Each side left gaps so that their patrols could get out.

No Man's Land – the land between the opposing trenches. Sometimes it was only 100 metres wide.

▲ **SOURCE H** A diagram of a typical British trench system

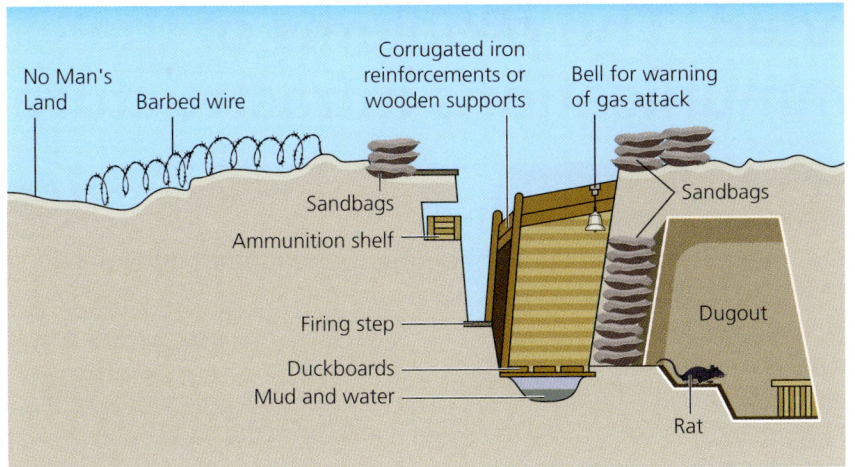

▲ SOURCE I A cross-section of a trench

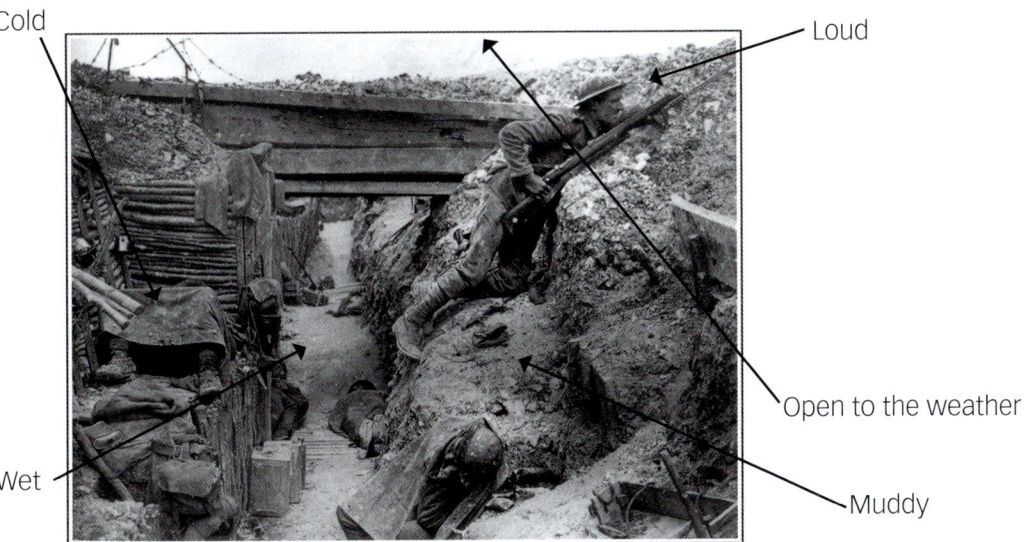

▲ SOURCE J British soldiers in a trench on the Western Front

Trench warfare

When most people think of the trenches, they think of troops going over the top to attack enemy trenches and suffering heavy losses. Trenches were protected by machine guns, heavy weapons which usually needed two or three men to operate them. They could fire between 400 and 500 bullets per minute. They were devastating against attacks by enemy troops. Machine guns were very effective defensive weapons but too heavy and difficult to use in attack.

Going over the top in a major attack was comparatively rare. Most of the work done in the trenches was routine. Infantry soldiers spent much of their time digging or repairing trenches or setting up barriers of barbed wire. They carted supplies and equipment up and down communications trenches. They spent long hours on sentry duty. Of course, it was still very dangerous. At any moment, a soldier could be killed by an enemy sniper or find himself on the end of an **artillery bombardment**. Artillery was by far the biggest cause of casualties in the war.

Helping the wounded: The problems of the transport and communications infrastructure

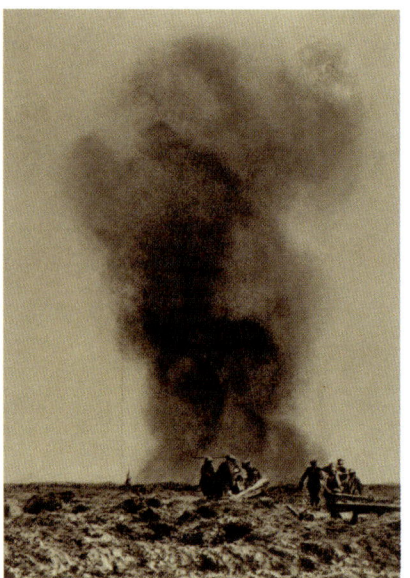

▲ **SOURCE K** A photograph from a British newspaper of 1917. The caption reads 'The British Advance: collecting wounded under fire. With a great shell bursting near them: a stretcher squad on No Man's Land picking up a wounded man.'

Research & Record

What were the challenges of helping the wounded on the Western Front?

Use the information on this page to complete the table that you started on page 112. Record the challenges that the Western Front posed to those trying to help the wounded in the First World War. You will be able to use these notes to answer the exam question on the page opposite.

Not surprisingly, the massive casualties and the churned-up landscapes after battles made it very difficult for the medical teams. They had to find the wounded, get them off the battlefield, get them assessed by a doctor to see what treatment they needed and then get them to a dressing station (see page 123) and then on to a hospital. The faster a wounded soldier was evacuated the better chance he had of surviving.

The first problem was locating injured soldiers and getting them back behind their own lines. The most seriously injured were usually out in No Man's Land. Stretcher bearers had to go out to the wounded, often in the dark and sometimes under fire.

Even when they reached their own lines it was difficult to move the wounded. Trenches were usually busy, packed with soldiers moving up and down and also equipment and weapons. Trenches were especially busy during an attack and this was obviously when there were the greatest number of wounded. Military rules also had a strict priority order. Top priority was given to the movement of ammunition, then to fighting troops, then to the wounded.

After they reached their **reserve trenches** there were still more challenges. There were ambulances to take the wounded away to hospitals or sometimes to trains or canal barges which would take them to hospitals further away. In a big battle, the ambulances could be overwhelmed by the sheer number of wounded. Another hazard was that the enemy often targeted communications trenches, roads and rail lines with artillery in order to disrupt communications. Roads were quickly cleared and patched up but they were uneven, and being bumped around must have been a nightmare for badly injured soldiers.

Apply ▶ Exam Practice

Question 1 style

Describe **one** feature of the problems involved in transporting wounded soldiers away from the battleground.

(4 marks)

Exam Tip

Describing features (Question 1)

1. Some students struggle with how to start their answer. Start your answer by **using the key phrase in the question**. This should help you to focus on the question as well as to get started.

2. Do not simply list a feature of the problems involved in transporting wounded soldiers away from the battleground. You need to **develop the feature** that you identify with some **description**.

Apply ▶ Exam Practice

Question 2a style

How useful are Sources L and M for an enquiry into the problems of transporting the wounded away from the battleground on the Western Front?

(8 marks)

> Our evacuation arrangements proved very satisfactory in spite of the **great difficulty caused by the long stretcher carry**. Each Battalion had a R.A.P. [Regimental Aid Post] behind its line in the forward area. **The RAP of the North Lancashire Regiment was very heavily shelled and eventually demolished**. The wounded were evacuated on motor ambulances. **Stretcher-bearers suffered very heavy casualties, one unit having 42 casualties out of 48**. All units have emphasised the excellent work of their Stretcher-Bearers.
>
> ▲ **SOURCE L** Extract from the War Diary of a British Field Hospital Unit August 1917. (War diaries like this were official military reports of activities in a day – or a few days. They are *not* the same as personal diaries.)

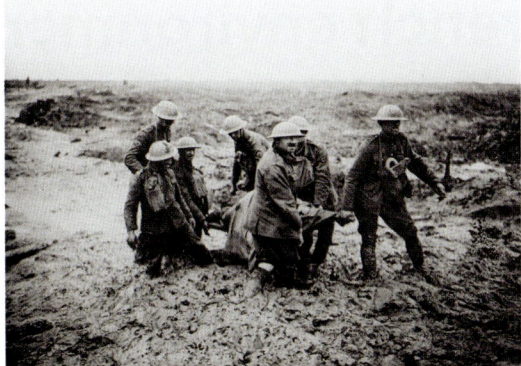

▲ **SOURCE M** A photograph from the National Army Museum showing stretcher bearers with a wounded soldier in 1917 near Ypres

Exam Tip

The usefulness of sources (Question 2a)

Your exam will include a source-based question.

- You have to analyse both sources carefully, identifying what they tell you and explaining why they are useful.
- You have just over ten minutes to answer this question in the exam. One paragraph for each source is enough for a high-level answer.
- You should focus on how they are useful for the enquiry in the question. The examiner does not want you to highlight problems with the sources. You could start, for example, *Source A is useful because it …*
- In the rest of your paragraph, develop and support your argument by referring to the content, the provenance and your wider knowledge of the enquiry.

C The content of the source

Before you begin to write, highlight/annotate the key information in the source, as we have in the example above for Source L.

K Your own knowledge of the period

You will need to bring in your own knowledge to explain how the source is useful for the enquiry in the question. Remember that:

- Stretcher bearers usually had to collect the wounded from No Man's Land. This was dangerous and often took place at night or under fire.
- During the Third Battle of Ypres there were 245,000 casualties, leading to the areas of treatment being very busy and slow.

P The provenance of the source

Remember that war diaries are official military reports. The source, therefore, gives us an excellent insight into the key information that was shared about the events and challenges experienced on the Western Front by a British Field Hospital unit in August 1917 when transporting the wounded.

Part 5 Conditions requiring medical treatment on the Western Front

The problems of ill health arising from the trench environment

Research & Record

What illnesses did soldiers experience as a result of the trench environment?

Use the information on these two pages to gather examples of both physical and psychological illnesses that were common in the trench environment.

Physical illnesses

- Trench fever – symptoms included headaches, sweating, painful joints, stomach problems
- .
- .

Psychological illnesses

- Shell shock – symptoms included tiredness, poor concentration, poor sleeping, violent shaking
- .
- .

Common illnesses on the Western Front

Even without any fighting, the simple fact that millions of men were gathered together in a relatively small area in difficult conditions was bound to lead to illness. We know a great deal about these problems because of the records kept by the British Army.

Trench fever

On the Western Front, there were thousands of men living in dirty, densely packed trenches. Disease was almost inevitable. Many Royal Army Medical Corps' (RAMC) records (see page 120) refer to a condition called Pyrexia of Unknown Origin (PUO). The soldiers usually called it trench fever. Historians estimate that around 20 to 30 per cent of all British troops suffered from it at some time. The symptoms were similar to influenza: headaches, sweating, painful joints and sometimes stomach problems. At first, doctors did not know what caused it. The notes of RAMC doctors show that by 1916 many of them suspected it was caused by lice, but this was not scientifically proven until 1918. Lice were a terrible problem in the trenches with so many men packed together. By 1918, bathing facilities and boiling and delousing uniforms helped to reduce the spread but the problem was never completely solved.

Trench foot

In many sectors of the Western Front there was a constant battle to stop trenches flooding with water, especially in winter. Trench foot was a horrible illness caused by soldiers standing in cold water and mud for long periods of time. Feet would swell, blister, go numb, turn red and eventually turn blue. In really bad cases, gangrene would set in. This meant that the tissue in the foot died and would have to be amputated. One British Army division reported that over 15 per cent of its men in January 1915 were suffering from trench foot. Soldiers were given water-resistant whale oil to put on their feet. The problem was only really solved with the introduction of waterproof rubber boots from about 1915 onwards but these were always in short supply.

Psychological injuries

As you have already read, life in the trenches was lived against a backdrop of artillery fire. Sometimes it was a distant thunder, other times soldiers would be under fire themselves. This could have a major psychological impact. Today we are much more aware of the causes and effects of mental health illnesses. We know that people can be scarred by difficult events, causing PTSD (Post Traumatic Stress Disorder). At the time of the war this was not well-understood. From quite early on, RAMC records show examples of soldiers experiencing psychological problems. The symptoms ranged from tiredness and poor concentration to poor sleeping, shaking violently and complete mental breakdown. Doctors used the term NYDN (Not Yet Diagnosed – Nervous) on their medical reports, but the condition was generally known as shell shock. Treatment was very basic and limited because there was so little understanding of the condition. The most serious cases were sent back to Britain to convalescent homes where they could get treatment. However, most soldiers were given a few days' rest and then returned to duty. There were around 80,000 recorded cases of shell shock but it seems likely that there were many more cases that were not recorded.

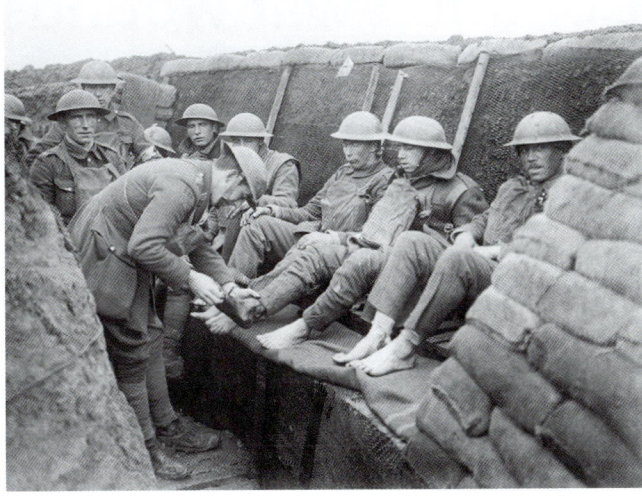

▲ **SOURCE N** RAMC doctor carrying out a foot inspection in a reserve trench in 1918

Patient went to France Aug 1914 with the original Expeditionary Force with the Royal Artillery. During the retreat from Mons, at Cambrai, on Aug. 27th they were nearly captured. German infantry surrounded them & were only 300 yards away. It is evident that the mental strain was considerable. At Ypres on April 1915 the explosion of a high-explosive shell lifted him from his feet & dashed him against the wheel of his field gun. He was dazed & semi-conscious for a short time. When he tried to talk to his comrades he found he could not speak. He was sent from hospital to hospital until 3 months later he regained speech but he has developed trembling in his limbs. His memory & intelligence are good. His organs are sound but the trembling makes him unfit for any duties.

▲ **SOURCE O** Medical notes for one soldier from June 1916. The soldier was eventually sent home in July 1916 as unfit for service

---

Apply ▶ Exam Practice

Question 1 style

Describe **one** feature of ill health among soldiers that arose from the trench environment. (4 marks)

Exam Tip

Describing features (Question 1)

Look again at the advice on how to approach this type of question on page 115.

Remember to:
- Identify a feature.
- Support the feature with some description.

Common war wounds on the Western Front

> ### Research & Record
>
> **What war wounds did soldiers experience due to the fighting on the Western Front?**
>
> While illness was a major problem, enemy fire was of course the main cause of injury and death on the Western Front. Complete the following two tasks using the information on pages 118–119.
>
> 1 Make a list of the nature of wounds from the type of weapon (for example, bullets – cut flesh, break bones, damage organs inside a soldier's body).
> 2 Use a table like this to record the problems and the solutions that were developed to deal with particular issues on the Western Front.
>
> | | Problems | Solution(s) developed |
> |---|---|---|
> | Head injuries | | |
> | Poison gas | | |
> | Infection | | |

The nature of wounds from the type of weapons

Different weapons caused different injuries.

Bullets

Rifle and machine gun bullets could smash through flesh and even break bones. Bullets often fragmented, breaking into pieces inside a soldier's body. According to an RAMC report based on the registers from Casualty Clearing Stations (CCS), bullets from rifles and machine guns caused about 39 per cent of casualties.

Artillery shells and shrapnel

Even more devastating than bullets were artillery shells. The RAMC report found that they caused around 58 per cent of casualties. A direct hit from high explosive shells would leave virtually no trace of a soldier's body. Soldiers had a deep and terrible fear of being blown to pieces and leaving no remains. Almost as deadly was shrapnel. Shrapnel shells exploded in the air and scattered razor-sharp pieces of metal at enormous speed.

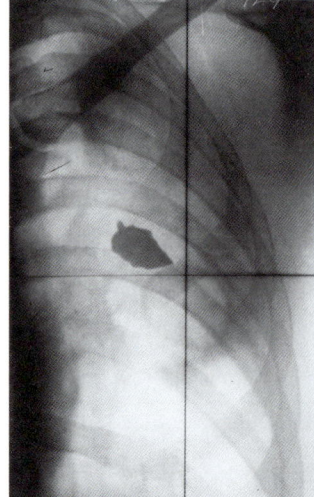

▲ SOURCE P X-rays taken by RAMC teams showing shrapnel wounds

Poison gas

Poison gas (chlorine) was first used by the Germans at the second Battle of Ypres in 1915. It proved quite successful in that it led to confusion and panic and allowed the Germans to advance. The British and their allies also used gas. There were three main types. Chlorine and phosgene attacked the lungs and could kill by suffocating a soldier. Mustard gas caused terrible burns on the eyes or skin. The main defence was the gas mask, which was rapidly introduced after the 1915 attack and was generally effective. Casualties from gas were relatively small compared to other weapons – around 6000 deaths, and most of those wounded by gas recovered. Doctors used oxygen cylinders to help victims breathe and most of those blinded recovered their sight in a few weeks. Despite this, gas had a major psychological impact, and it was greatly feared by the soldiers.

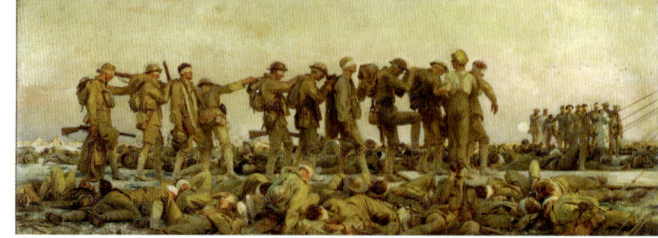

▲ SOURCE Q A painting by the war artist John Singer Sergeant showing soldiers who had been blinded by gas

Problems with treating the wounds from weapons of war

The power of the new weaponry meant that wounds were deeper and more severe than in previous wars. The scale of the fighting and the intensity of gun and artillery fire meant that all parts of the body were likely to be hit. There were over 270,000 cases of wounds to arms and legs. Over 41,000 men had arms or legs amputated. There were also massive numbers of head and eye wounds – over 60,000 in total. At the start of the war, soldiers only had cloth caps but the Army quickly introduced the steel Brodie helmet in 1915. It was estimated that the helmet reduced the number of fatal head wounds by around 80 per cent.

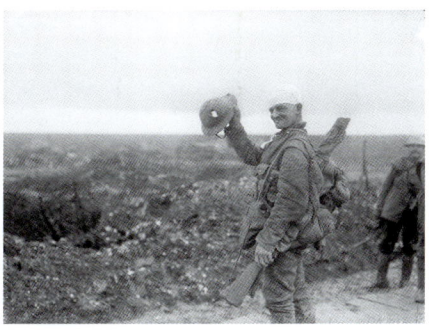

▲ **SOURCE R** A wounded British soldier at the Somme in 1916, showing off the helmet which probably saved him from a shrapnel shell

Blood loss

As well as the actual wounds themselves, the medical teams faced the obvious problem that the wounded were usually in a churned-up landscape which was being fired on. The wounded often had to wait for long periods of time before they were found and treated, and many died from the loss of blood from their wounds.

Infection

Infection was also a major problem, and at first it was made worse by the medical thinking of the day. The RAMC assumed that dressings would keep soldiers free of infection long enough for them to be transported back to hospitals. But they were wrong. The number of casualties was very high and so it took longer to transport the wounded for treatment. Also, the farmlands of the Western Front had been treated with manure to make crops grow. The side effect of this was that there were many bacteria in the soil and these bacteria caused infection. The two main types of infection were tetanus and **gas gangrene**. Gangrene set in when the blood flow to a part of the body was cut off. Gas gangrene infected the gangrenous area and caused bubbles of gas under the skin. It was deadly and spread quickly through the body, potentially killing within 24 hours.

The RAMC recognised the problems and tried to react. Tetanus was largely solved by giving all the wounded an anti-tetanus injection. Gas gangrene proved much more difficult to tackle. In 1915, they started treating the wounds at the Casualty Clearing Stations, cutting away infected tissue and applying antiseptics. This improved the survival rate, but deaths remained high until surgery moved closer to the front line (see page 123).

Apply ▶ Exam Practice

Question 1 style

Describe **one** feature of the nature of the wounds caused by the fighting on the Western Front. (2 marks)

Describe **one** feature of the effects of gas attacks on the Western Front. (2 marks)

Part 5 Medical treatment on the Western Front

> ### Research & Record
>
> **What work was carried out by the RAMC and nurses on the Western Front?**
>
> The medical care of soldiers on the Western Front was carried out by men and women in the Royal Army Medical Corps (RAMC) and nurses.
>
> Use the information on these two pages to gather examples of their work under both headings. You may also want to look back at previous pages and sources, for example Source N on page 117.
>
> *RAMC*
> - Foot inspections for trench foot
> -
> -
>
> *Nurses*
> - Drove motor ambulances
> -
> -

Royal Army Medical Corps

The work of planning for the medical needs on the Western Front, recruiting enough medical staff and actually treating the troops was the job of the RAMC. When war broke out in 1914, the RAMC estimated that they would need 12,000 doctors. Most of these were recruited from Britain's population of civilian doctors. This was an area of success for the British military, which was helped by the fact that many doctors volunteered even before they were called up. This became more systematic through the war. From 1915, the War Office could call up any doctor under the age of 45. Doctors were recruited, trained and replaced throughout the war and by 1918 the RAMC had around 13,000 medical officers. However, the doctors were only part of a huge operation. By the end of the war, there were over 150,000 men and women involved in medical care. As well as doctors, this included nurses, stretcher bearers, ambulance and train drivers and many others.

Nurses

Queen Alexandra's Imperial Military Nursing Service

In 1914, the British Army had around 300 (female) nurses of the Queen Alexandra's Imperial Military Nursing Service (QAIMNS). This was formed in 1902 and was made up of highly trained and qualified nurses. In the initial stages of the war, the Army was reluctant to let nurses near the front line. However, this attitude changed by 1915–16 as the scale of the casualties became clear and meant that many more nurses were needed. Attitudes also changed as the treatment of the wounded adapted to the conditions of the Western Front.

First Aid Nursing Yeomanry

Many of the extra nurses were provided by the First Aid Nursing Yeomanry (FANY). This organisation of volunteer nurses was founded in 1907 by a former British soldier who hoped it would provide fast responses and treatment to men wounded on the battlefield. In the initial stages of the war, the British Army did not want to make use of them, but they persevered and by 1916 the FANY were a key element of the medical care for British troops on the Western Front. They drove ambulances, and provided mobile kitchens and bathing facilities. They helped to evacuate the wounded from the battlefields, often under fire – the FANY were awarded almost 40 medals for bravery by the British and French governments. The FANY were particularly well-respected and highly prized for the bravery and ability in driving motor ambulances, and maintaining and repairing the ambulances which often broke down. FANY nurses also provided staff for Regimental Aid Depots (RADs) and provided many of the staff who ran the British military hospitals.

> **Apply — Exam Practice**
>
> **Question 1 style**
>
> 1. Describe **one** feature of the work of the Royal Army Medical Corps (RAMC) on the Western Front. (2 marks)
> 2. Describe **one** feature of the work of nurses on the Western Front. (2 marks)

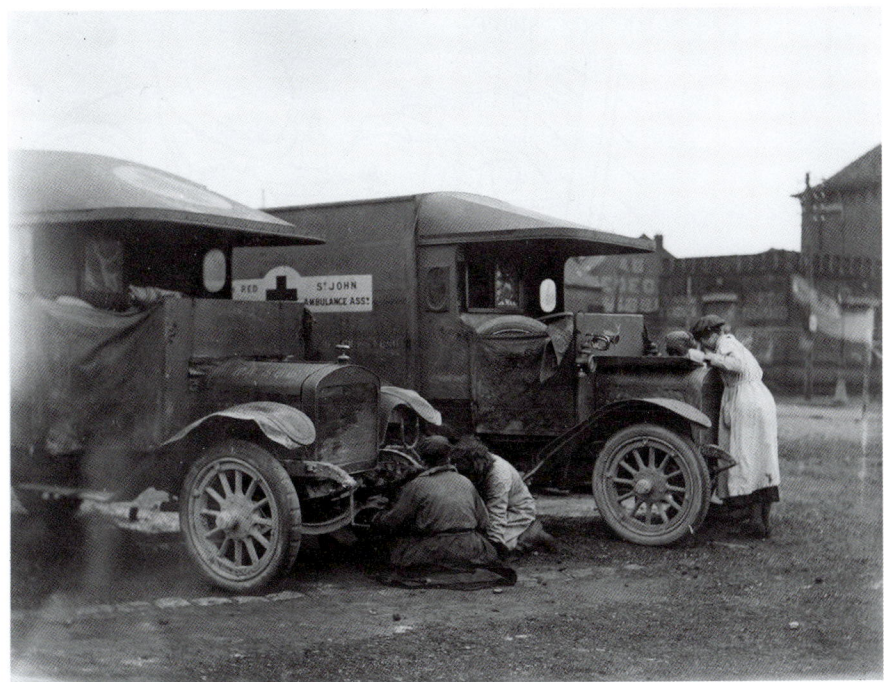

◀ **SOURCE S** Nurses carrying out repairs on their motor ambulances at St Omer, around 1917

Transport and the stages of treatment on the Western Front

> ### Research & Record
>
> **Where were the wounded cared for and treated on the Western Front?**
>
> Use pages 122–123 to complete your own copy of a table like this. Record details of the transport used and the treatment carried out at each stage on the British sector of the Western Front.
>
> | Stage of treatment | Details of the transport used to get the wounded to the stage | Details of the treatment carried out |
> |---|---|---|
> | Regimental Aid Posts (RAPs) | | |
> | Casualty Clearing Stations (CCS) | | |
> | Dressing stations | | |
> | Base hospitals | | |

Transporting the wounded

Throughout the war, the priority for the RAMC was to get the wounded out of the line of fire and to a medical officer. For a soldier who could not walk, the first stage of the process was usually the stretcher bearer. They carried supplies to give basic first aid, such as bandages and morphine for pain relief. There were usually about 16 stretcher bearers to a unit of 1000 men so in a battle they often struggled to cope with the numbers of casualties. Stretcher bearers usually took the wounded to a Regimental Aid Post (RAP).

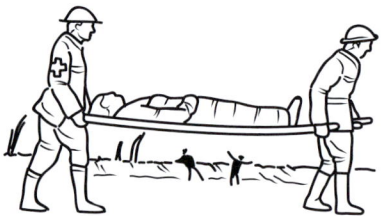

In the early stages of the war, the British Army only had horse-drawn ambulances. These were slow and under-powered and the horses needed a lot of looking after. By 1915, the Army was replacing horse-drawn ambulances with motor ambulances. Motor ambulances often got stuck in the mud, and so the use of horse-drawn ambulances continued. Ambulances took casualties straight to hospital, or they might offload them on to trains or barges. This has been described as the worst aspect of being seriously wounded because of the pain caused by being transported.

Stages of treatment: The chain of evacuation

Regimental Aid Posts

Regimental Aid Posts (RAPs) were usually close to the front line, in a support or communication trench or perhaps in a building (or the ruins of a building). Their role was to patch up troops so they could return to duty as quickly as possible. There was usually one Medical Officer (MO) or orderlies trained to give first aid. If the wounded soldier could not be treated here then he was moved to the next stage.

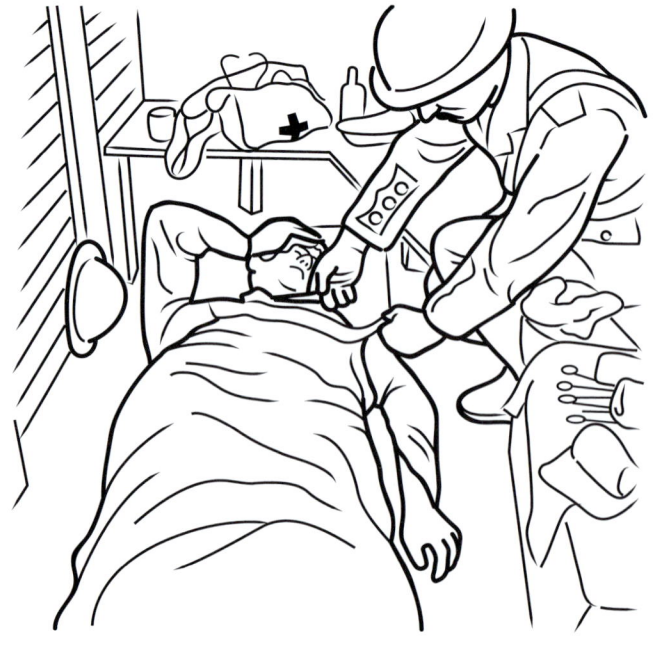

Field hospital and dressing stations

A field hospital was a mobile unit of the RAMC with an MO, orderlies and sometimes nurses. The field hospital ran dressing stations, often set up in a tent or a building or ruin, usually about 400–500 metres from the trenches. Dressing stations could treat around 150 men at full capacity. They treated light wounds but the main job of this unit was sorting out the wounded into the most urgent, serious cases and cases that were less serious and could return to duty. From here, the wounded were taken to Casualty Clearing Stations.

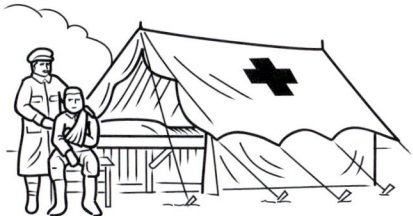

Casualty Clearing Stations

The Casualty Clearing Station (CCS) was the first major medical facility that a wounded soldier would reach. A CCS might be set up in tents, but the RAMC also used schools, factories or other buildings.

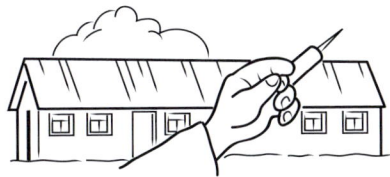

When the war began, CCSs were usually around 10 miles behind the fighting and their main role was triage (sorting). They sorted the wounded into categories:

- Return to duty with minor treatment and rest
- Immediate treatment
- Transport to base hospitals for treatment
- No chance of recovery

The RAMC discovered that the quicker the treatment the better the chance of survival, so CCSs gradually moved closer to the front line and became more like small hospitals. As well as medical staff, orderlies and nurses, they had operating theatres and they made use of the latest technology like mobile X-ray machines (see page 127). Emergency operations could be performed at CCSs, and they could handle around 1000 casualties at full capacity. If soldiers needed time to recover, or if they needed more specialist treatment, they went to the next stage, the base hospital.

Base hospitals

Base hospitals could be existing hospitals, or they could be set up in buildings taken over by the RAMC. Base hospitals were modern, fully equipped hospitals with modern technologies. The larger hospitals could treat around 2500 at any one time. In the early stages of the war, they dealt with the serious cases. However, as the CCSs evolved to take on more of these cases, the base hospitals took on the role of caring for the wounded after their treatment and in many cases preparing the wounded to be transferred back to Britain.

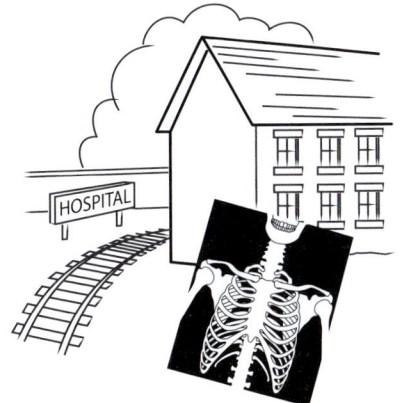

The underground hospital at Arras

The RAMC were always looking for ways to improve treatment. One of the most remarkable achievements was the underground base hospital at Arras (see page 111). It could treat around 700 soldiers at any one time. It had running water, electricity and operating theatres and by 1917 it had all the latest medical technology such as X-rays. It was run extremely effectively with stretcher bearers, orderlies, nurses, doctors and all the other medical staff working together as a team. During the Battle of Arras in April 1917 there were over 7000 casualties but the hospital coped with them all and was never overwhelmed, despite being hit by German artillery which disrupted water and power supplies.

The work of the RAMC and nurses exam practice

Apply ▶ Exam Practice

Question 2a style

How useful are Sources T and U for an enquiry into the work of medical staff on the Western Front? Explain your answer using Sources T and U and your knowledge of the historical context. (8 marks)

My problem in a battle was to keep all the surgeons busy with cases really urgently needing operation. Every case was brought in, put on the table, his wounds undone and a decision made, by me, as to what happened to him, either to the resuscitation ward, to the preoperation ward, to a ward especially kept for the dying, straight to one of the surgical wards or for immediate evacuation. At the same time I had not to send so many to the pre-operating room that the last case would have to wait longer for his operation than if sent to the base; and, above all, not to send cases in for operation so badly wounded as to be unlikely to recover. It was a fairly difficult business.

▲ **SOURCE T** Description of the work of an RAMC officer in a Casualty Clearing Station in 1916

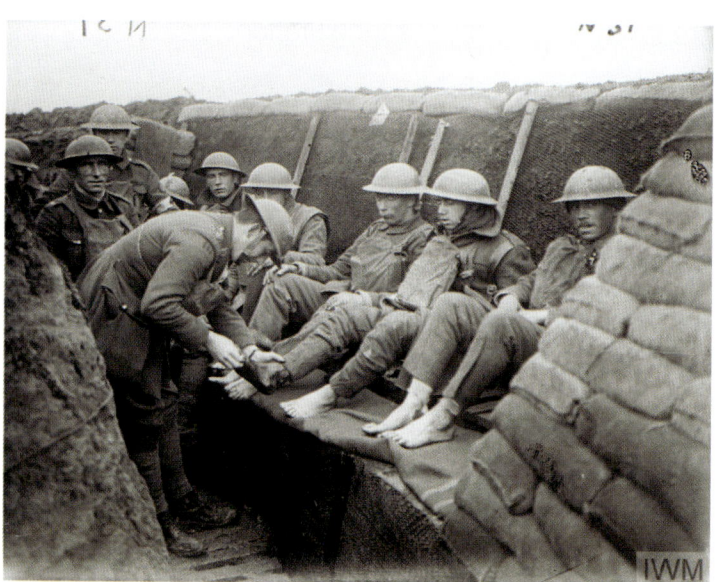

▲ **SOURCE U** An RAMC doctor carrying out a foot inspection in a reserve trench in 1918

Exam Tip

The usefulness of sources (Question 2a)

Remind yourself of the CKP advice on page 115 about how to approach this type of question.

C Look carefully at the **content** of the sources. Explain what we can learn from the sources about the work of medical staff on the Western Front.

K Use your contextual **knowledge**. Source T describes the decisions that an RAMC officer made in a Casualty Clearing Station about the treatment that the wounded would receive for their injuries. Source U shows us that RAMC doctors also went out into the trenches to inspect soldiers' feet and try to avoid further cases of trench foot. Can you remember who the RAMC were? Who else gave medical treatment on the Western Front? If you can't, look back at page 120 before you plan your answer.

P Use the **provenance** of the source. Explain why the nature/author of the source is useful for this enquiry and link to the **content**. Source T is written by an RAMC officer and it will be useful for this enquiry because the author describes the work that he did in a Casualty Clearing Station following a battle when it was very busy. His description of the decisions he had to make are useful for understanding how an RAMC officer had to work under pressure to decide the best treatment for each injured soldier.

Exam Tip

Use connectives and evidence for stronger arguments

When explaining how a source is useful for an enquiry, you have to prove that the source is useful. For example:

Source T is useful for an enquiry into the work of medical staff because it shows us the RAMC officer made important decisions following a battle about the treatment that would be given to each injured soldier. The source is useful as it tells us that the RAMC officer prioritised those injured who urgently needed treatment when he writes 'my problem in a battle was to keep all the surgeons busy with cases really urgently needing operation.' He goes on to describe the system of triage that operated in a Casualty Clearing Station when he lists the options available to him as 'his wounds undone and a decision made, by me, as to what happened to him …' for each wounded soldier. This tells us that an RAMC officer had to make important decisions that would determine the future of each wounded soldier. The nature of Source T is useful for an enquiry into the work of the RAMC because it is a first-hand account written by an officer who served in a Casualty Clearing Station during a busy battle of 1916, possibly the Battle of the Somme. His first-hand account gives us an insight into how an RAMC officer had to remain as calm as possible to work under pressure and make decisions about the treatment received including immediate surgery, evacuation or to a ward for the dying.

Use connectives to link your arguments to the enquiry

Phrases like 'is useful for an enquiry into', 'this tells us' and 'this shows' are called connectives because they link your arguments to the enquiry and so help you prove how the source is useful.

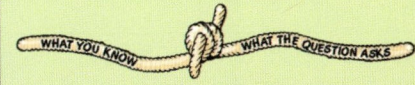

Add specific knowledge

Provide evidence to substantiate (support) your argument.

Apply ▶ Exam Practice

Use the Exam Tip to write a paragraph explaining how useful Source U is for an enquiry into the work of medical staff. Remember to:
- Explain how the content and/or the provenance of the source is useful.
- Develop your explanation with some of your own contextual knowledge.

Apply ▶ Exam Practice

Question 2b style

Use the Exam Tip on page 133 to help you answer this question:

How could you follow up Source U to find out more about the work of medical staff on the Western Front? (4 marks)

Detail in Source U that I would follow up: _____

Question I would ask: _____

What type of source I could use: _____

How this might help answer my question: _____

Part 5 The significance of the Western Front for experiments in surgery and medicine

Research & Record

How did surgery and medicine advance on the Western Front during the First World War?

The type of wounds and problems with treating them during the First World War brought about important developments in areas such as surgery, plastic surgery, treating burns, treating head and brain injuries, fighting infection and the challenge of blood loss.

Use the information on pages 126–129 to complete your own copy of this bingo card.

Experiments in surgery and medicine bingo		
What was the Carrel–Dakin method?	**Why** was gas gangrene a problem on the Western Front?	**What** was the Thomas splint?
What impact did the Thomas splint have on the treatment of leg wounds?	**What** were the problems with using X-ray machines on the Western Front?	**How** were the problems with X-ray machines overcome during the years of the war?
How was plastic surgery developed during the First World War?	**What** developments changed the approach to head wounds and brain injuries?	**What** developments led to more successful blood transfusions on the battlefield?

The treatment of infection

By 1914 aseptic surgery was well advanced (see page 67) but it was not possible in battlefield conditions or even in crowded, dirty dressing stations. The most serious problem by far though was gas gangrene (see page 119) which was deadly and spread quickly through the body, potentially killing within 24 hours. Gas gangrene bacteria was in the soil so as blasts or bullet wounds drove dirt and bits of uniform into wounds, the bacteria for infection was already present in the body by the time the wounded arrived for treatment.

At first, medical staff returned to antiseptic techniques, spraying wounds with antiseptics like carbolic acid. But this was painful and not very effective. Many surgeons found that they had little or no choice but to amputate limbs to stop the spread of infection. The problem of gas gangrene was never completely overcome, but doctors were constantly experimenting and trying new methods. Just as importantly, they were writing articles in journals which other doctors were able to read and this encouraged further experimentation.

One helpful development came in 1915 when the respected scientist Sir Almroth Wright proposed the use of a saline solution to clean wounds. This did help to reduce infections. A more effective approach was the Carrel–Dakin method (named after the two doctors who developed it in 1917, Alexis Carrel and Henry Dakin). This involved putting tubes carrying a chemical called sodium hypochlorite into wounds. This killed bacteria, and was therefore very effective at fighting gas gangrene. However, it was a complicated treatment. It needed the constant supervision of a medic and was often impossible in battlefield conditions.

The biggest advance in fighting gas gangrene was the policy of shifting surgery closer to the front line, either in field hospitals or CCSs. This meant the wounded were operated on earlier, allowing surgeons to cut away tissues around wounds which had been contaminated by soil or clothing. This was called **excision**. It prevented gas gangrene and other infections like tetanus from infecting wounded soldiers.

The treatment of leg wounds: The Thomas splint

From the start of the war there were very high numbers of serious leg wounds from bullets, shrapnel and explosions. In the early stages of the war, serious leg injuries tended to be fatal – there was a survival rate of only about 20 percent if major bones were broken. This was because when wounded soldiers tried to move, their broken bones would move and cause damage inside the leg, leading to internal bleeding. Soldiers mostly died from blood loss or shock.

The solution to this problem was the Thomas splint which was invented by the Liverpool surgeon Hugh Owen Thomas and used across the Western Front from 1916. The Thomas splint stabilised an injured leg so that the broken bones did not do more damage. This usually helped to prevent blood loss. This in turn meant that the wounded soldier was strong enough to have surgery at the CCS, which greatly improved his chances.

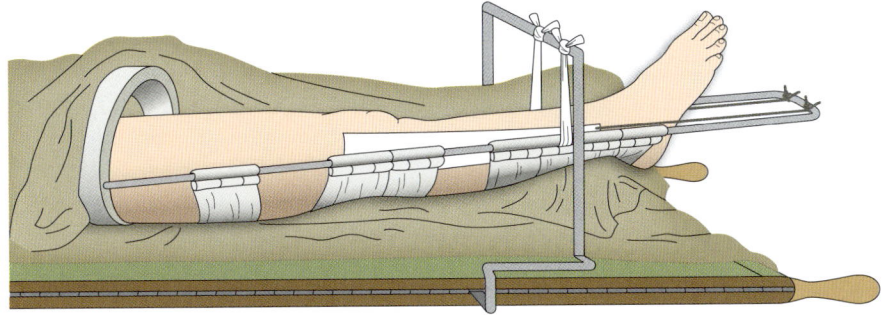

▲ **SOURCE V** The Thomas splint in use

Mobile X-ray units

Doctors realised early on how useful X-rays could be for detecting shrapnel or bullets in a wounded soldier's body. Knowing the location of a fragment of metal made it much easier for the surgeon to remove it.

In the early stages of the war the RAMC only had two X-ray machines but the government ordered more as soon as it became clear how useful they were. By 1916, most CCSs and hospitals had X-ray machines. There were still problems, however. The machines were large and delicate and broke down or overheated easily. Medics tried to solve this problem by using machines in a rota, allowing one machine to cool down while another was in use. Another problem was that X-ray prints were on glass plates and the plates were fragile. A big breakthrough here was the invention of celluloid film for creating prints.

Treatment with X-rays improved still further as the technology developed to make them more mobile. As you have seen, the RAMC realised that it was more effective to have treatment available close to the front line and the new X-ray machines made it easier for them to move along with the CCSs as the fighting moved.

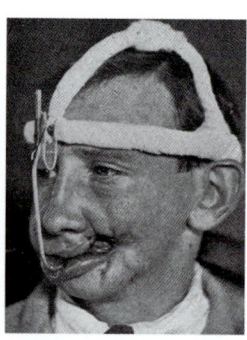
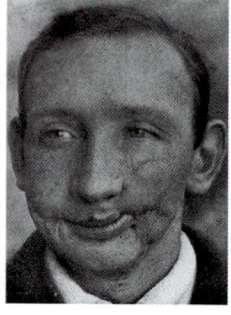
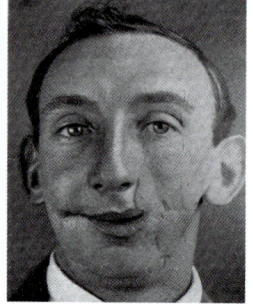

▲ **SOURCE W** Photographs showing the reconstruction of a soldier's face, from a 1920 report by Harold Gillies

Plastic surgery

Plastic surgery had been carried out centuries earlier, but it was limited by the danger of infection and pain. With these two problems solved, surgeons could begin to repair some of the terrible wounds caused in war by bullets and shrapnel.

Improvements in the First World War

Surgeons carried out over 11,000 plastic surgery operations, increasing their experience and learning from each other. By November 1915, seven hospitals in France had specialist departments for dealing with wounds needing plastic surgery, particularly to the face and head.

Surgeons developed new techniques using jaw splints, wiring and metal plates as 'replacement' cheeks. Another major improvement was the use of skin grafts, taking skin from another part of the patient's body and grafting it on to the area of the wound.

Harold Gillies, a New Zealand surgeon serving in France, persuaded the army's chief surgeon that a specialist facial injury care unit was needed in England for the wounded. In 1917, The Queen's Hospital was opened in Kent, specialising in repairing facial injuries.

Treating head and brain injuries

During the early years of the war, soldiers also experienced a high number of head and brain injuries. One major reason was that for soldiers standing in trenches, their heads were the most vulnerable part of their bodies. Little was known about the brain and so head injuries were not operated on in 1914. It would have taken a long time to operate on a head wound and so injuries were simply bandaged.

The number of head and brain injuries forced surgeons to try new ideas. Two developments changed the approach to head wounds and particularly brain surgery:

- Blood transfusions and saline solutions reduced shock and so soldiers were fit enough to cope with operations on their head.
- The large numbers of head wounds enabled surgeons to improve their skills and develop new techniques for operating on head wounds. The use of X-rays enabled surgeons to locate, identify and remove bullet and shell fragments and the surgeon Harvey Cushing invented a surgical magnet to extract bullets from head wounds.

Blood transfusions and blood banks

You have already seen many references in this section to the problem of blood loss. Serious injuries almost always led to major blood loss, and this in turn could cause a patient to go into shock and die soon afterwards. The answer to this problem was blood transfusions (see page 109).

The problem of blood clotting

One problem with transfusions was that they could only be performed by attaching the patient to a blood donor. It was not possible to store blood because it clotted and became too thick to be given to the patient. The first step to solving the problem was the discovery that the chemical sodium citrate could help prevent blood from clotting. This treatment was developed by doctors in several different countries, but it was widespread in the USA and Canada. In 1915, a Canadian doctor serving with British forces called Bruce Robertson introduced a system of taking blood from donors in large bottles, adding sodium citrate and filtering it to remove clots. This meant that transfusions could be carried out much more easily from the bottles, without a tube connecting patient and donor.

Blood transfusion on the battlefield

There were other important developments by other doctors. In 1915, the RAMC doctor Geoffrey Keynes developed a portable transfusion kit which was small enough to be carried and used on the front line. It had a filtering system to prevent clotting. It was very effective, but the blood supply had to be constantly changed to keep it fresh. In the same year, the American doctor Richard Weil discovered that if blood treated with sodium citrate was refrigerated it would keep for several days.

The blood bank at Cambrai

In 1916, two researchers in the USA, Francis Rous and James Turner, discovered that adding a citrate glucose solution to blood meant that it could last for several weeks. When the USA entered the war in 1917, the American doctor Oswald Hope Robertson (no relation to Bruce Robertson) was posted to serve at a British CCS near Cambrai. Robertson adopted all the developments he had seen in blood transfusion and added his own. He took blood which had been treated with citrate glucose, filtered it and stored it in two-litre bottles, which he stored in ammunition boxes packed in with sawdust and ice. He stored only blood group O because it was compatible with almost all other blood types and would not need testing.

Hope Robertson had effectively created the first blood bank, and it saved many soldiers wounded at the Battle of Cambrai in 1917. He ran training courses to share his methods, and he and others continued to experiment and innovate. Better refrigeration allowed larger stocks of blood to be held. The RAMC also started keeping records of the blood types of soldiers so that they knew which blood type to give.

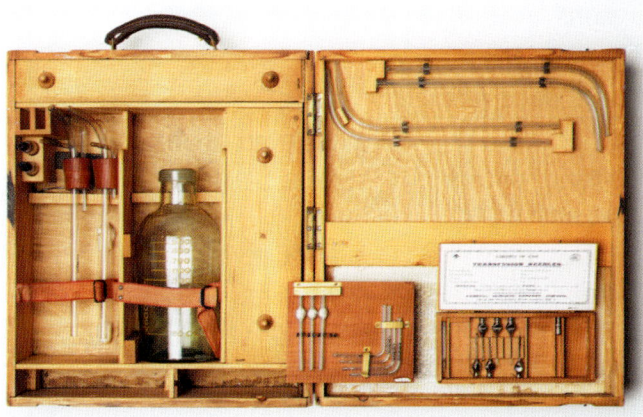

▲ **SOURCE X** The portable transfusion kit developed by Geoffrey Keynes

Summarise

Can you remember what these visuals help you to recall?

1.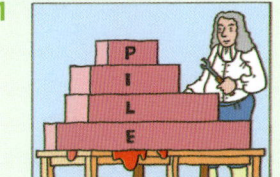
2.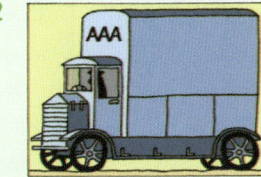

3. Use the memory aid below to explain how each of these Bs helped to overcome the problem of blood loss.

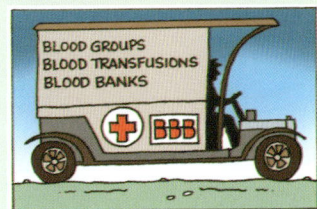

Part 5 The British sector of the Western Front, 1914–18: injuries, treatment and the trenches period review

Review

What illnesses and injuries did soldiers experience on the Western Front and how were these treated?

Fill in a table like the one below to review the period. This table has been started to give you some ideas.

Theme	Conditions on the Western Front leading to illness or injury	Individuals	Treatments
The British sector of the Western Front	Constant fire and shelling on No Man's Land Narrow trenches Muddy terrain		
The work of RAMC and nurses	Trench foot Trench fever Bullet and shrapnel wounds Head injuries Effects of gas attacks Gas gangrene		Change of socks Whale oil
Medical treatment on the Western Front		Volunteer medical professionals Doctors Surgeons Medical orderlies Ambulance drivers	
The system of transport and treatment areas on the Western Front		Stretcher bearers Ambulance drivers (horse-drawn and motor) Medical professionals (see above)	Chain of evacuation First aid at a Regimental Aid Post Casualty Clearing Station Base hospital Underground hospital at Arras
New techniques in surgery and medicine		Alexis Carrel Henry Dakin Harvey Cushing	Carrel–Dakin method Thomas splint Facial reconstruction Blood bank at Cambrai

> **Revision Tip**
>
> When you revise for the historic environment section of your exam, make sure you can describe the features of all injuries, treatments and the conditions in the trenches on the Western Front.

Apply ▶ Recall Challenges

1 Know the key developments

a Why were motor ambulances used on the Western Front?
b How did the blood bank improve the treatment of the wounded during the Battle of Cambrai?
c What impact did the Thomas splint have on soldiers' leg injuries?
d What problem on the battlefield did the Carrel–Dakin method overcome, and how?
e How did mobile X-ray machines improve the treatment of injuries on the Western Front?

2 Know the historical sources

Make an A4 copy of this bingo card. You will need plenty of space to write in each box.

Historical sources bingo		
Hospital records from a base hospital in Ypres	Diary from a stretcher bearer during 1917	Royal Army Medical Corps records from the Battle of the Somme in 1916
A national newspaper in 1916	An article in the medical journal *The Lancet* in 1918	A photograph of injured soldiers waiting outside a Casualty Clearing Station in 1917

a For each historical source, from memory, describe the information that is likely to be included. Then check your answers with your teacher.
b For each historical source, explain how it would be useful for an enquiry into the injuries sustained and treatments used on the British sector of the Western Front.

Apply ▶ Exam Practice

Question 1 style

1a Describe **one** feature of the treatment given to the wounded at a Dressing Station on the Western Front. (2 marks)

1b Describe **one** feature of the treatment given to the wounded at a Casualty Clearing Station on the Western Front. (2 marks)

Apply ▶ Exam Practice

Question 2a and 2b style

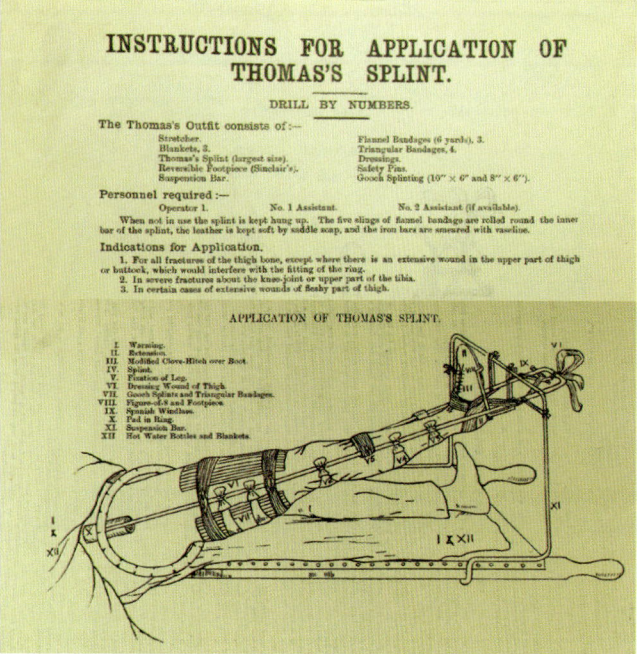

▲ **SOURCE Y** A training manual showing how to use the Thomas splint

It is absolutely essential for success that excision should be done as soon as possible after receiving a wound because in such cases gas gangrene may become widely spread within 24 hours. It is therefore necessary to operate on such cases before the patient is sent by train to the base hospital. This method of treatment has entirely replaced the application of strong antiseptics to a recent wound, or the use of continual saline infusions. It is a method whose value is agreed upon by the surgeons of all the Allies, and has recently been unanimously approved by the Meeting of the Surgeons of the Allied Armies in Paris.

▲ **SOURCE Z** Senior RAMC officer, Sir Anthony Bowlby, speaking in 1917 to a committee of MPs about medical care in the trenches

2a How useful are Sources Y and Z for an enquiry into new techniques being used on the Western Front to deal with injuries?
Explain your answer, using Sources Y and Z and your knowledge of the historical context. (8 marks)

2b How could you follow up Source Z to find out more about new techniques being used on the Western Front to deal with injuries?

In your answer, you must give the question you would ask and the type of source you could use. (4 marks)

Detail in Source AA that I would follow up:
_____

Question I would ask:
_____

What type of source I could use:
_____

How this might help answer my question:
_____

Exam Tip

Follow-up enquiry from a source (Question 2b)

Your exam will include a question that asks you to plan a follow-up enquiry from one of the two sources provided.

Look at the steps below that explain how to answer the following question:

How could you follow up Source T (page 124) to find out more about the work of the RAMC on the Western Front? (4 marks)

Steps	Possible answer
Select a **detail from the source**. This should be a quotation from a written source or something you can see in a visual source.	Detail in Source T (page 124) that I would follow up: 'keep all the surgeons busy with cases really urgently needing operation'.
Write a **question** that is **linked to the detail above** and would enable you to find out more about the enquiry in the question.	Question I would ask: What operations did surgeons of the RAMC carry out in a Casualty Clearing Station?
Select a **contemporary source** that will give you the answer to your question. Make it **specific** to the Western Front.	What type of source I could use: Royal Army Medical Corps medical records from a Casualty Clearing Station on the Western Front in 1916.
Explain how the source you have chosen will answer your question.	How this might help answer my question: These records will contain details of the operations carried out by RAMC surgeons in the Casualty Clearing Station during a battle.

Exam Tip

The usefulness of sources (Question 2a)

Look again at the advice on how to approach this type of question on page 115.

Remember to focus on why the source is useful and to use your knowledge of the focus of the enquiry.

- Consider what the content of each source tells us about the new techniques being used on the Western Front.
- How can you develop this using your own contextual knowledge?
- Consider how the nature (type of source) makes the provenance of the source useful for this enquiry.

Exam Tip

Follow-up enquiry from a source (Question 2b)

Look again at the advice on how to approach this type of question on page 125.

Remember to focus all parts of your answer on the enquiry in the question.

- Select a quotation from Source AA (page 132).
- Write a closed question that will give you more information about the new techniques being used on the Western Front.
- Select a specific contemporary source that will have the answer to your question.
- Explain how your source will answer your question.

Glossary

almhouses a house, founded by a charity, offering accommodation for poor people.

amputate to cut off a part of the body (often a limb) by surgery

amulet a charm that the wearer believes gives protection from disease

anaesthetic pain relief, usually through drugs

anatomy the science of understanding the structure and make-up of the body

antibiotic type of drug that is capable of fighting bacterial infection

antiseptic surgery surgery during which infection is avoided usually by killing germs with chemicals

apothecary a person who prepared and sold medicines

artillery bombardment heavy and concentrated attack from a large number of powerful guns

aseptic surgery surgery during which infection is avoided by preventing it happening, e.g. by sterilising instruments

astrology the study of the planets and how they might influence the lives of people

barber surgeon a barber who would perform minor surgery of wounds, bloodletting and extracting teeth alongside the cutting of hair

bleeding or **bloodletting** the treatment of opening a vein or applying leeches to draw blood from the patient

blood transfusion taking (compatible) blood from one person and giving it to another, usually because of blood lost through injury

buboes black swellings in the armpits and groin that were symptoms of the Black Death

capillaries tiny blood vessels that connect arteries and veins

carbolic spray used during surgical operations to kill germs in the air around the operating table

cesspool a place for collecting and storing sewage

chemotherapy treatment of a disease such as cancer by the use of chemicals

cholera an infection that causes severe watery diarrhoea (it often results from drinking dirty water)

clots formed when blood dries, usually outside the human body

compound something made up of two or more elements

creeping barrage artillery tactic in which guns fire just ahead of advancing troops

cure-all a medicine usually sold for a profit. In the nineteenth century they were often made from a mix of ingredients that had no medical benefits

dissection the cutting up and examination of a body

DNA deoxyribonucleic acid, the molecule that genes are made of

dysentery a severe infection causing frequent, fluid bowel movements

endoscope an instrument used to view inside the body

epidemic a sudden, widespread appearance of an infectious disease

excision surgical removal by cutting

gangrene type of infection

gas gangrene a lethal infection that caused bubbles of gas under the skin

genes microscopic parts of humans and animals which determine characteristics, e.g. hair colour

herbal remedies a treatment for illness using herbs

infectious capable of spreading

inoculation technique that involves giving patients small doses of disease to build up their defences

keyhole surgery surgical operation performed through a very small incision, using special instruments and an endoscope

laissez-faire belief that governments should not interfere in people's lives

leprosy a contagious disease that affects the skin and nerves

ligatures threads used to tie a blood vessel during an operation

magic bullets pills made from chemicals that kill particular infections inside the body

miasma smells from decomposing material that were believed to cause disease

microbe a tiny single-celled living organism too small to be seen by the naked eye

microorganisms organisms like germs that can only be seen under a microscope

microscope an instrument that allows the viewing of very small objects

MRSA methicillin-resistant staphylococcus aureus – bacteria that can cause infections in different parts of the body and is resistant to antibiotics

National Insurance a system that gives workers medical help and sick pay if they cannot work through illness

paediatrics branch of medicine specialising in children and young people

pasteurisation process of heating that destroys harmful bacteria

penicillin the first antibiotic drug, produced from the mould penicillium, used to treat infections

pharmaceutical industry large businesses that mass-produce drugs for medicine and healthcare

physician a person qualified to diagnose and recommend treatment for disease and illness

physiology the study of how the body works

purging removing any leftover food from the digestive system

quinine the drug treatment for malaria

radiation a form of energy in a wave form

radiation therapy or radiotherapy, treatment of a disease, such as cancer, by the use of X-rays or similar forms of radiation

reserve trenches trenches where troops were stationed if they needed to support front line trenches

scarlet fever a contagious bacterial infection

septum a wall separating the right and left hand sides of the heart

smallpox a serious infectious disease that causes skin blemishes and death. This was eradicated in the 1970s through vaccination programmes.

spontaneous generation the theory that decaying matter turns into germs

staphylococcus bacteria found on the skin that can cause infection if the bacteria become trapped

sterilise to destroy all living microorganisms from surfaces and surgical instruments

sulphonamide an antibacterial drug used to treat bronchitis and pneumonia

supernatural something that cannot be given an ordinary explanation

superstition an unreasonable belief based on ignorance and sometimes fear

transplant an operation in which tissue or organs is moved from one part of the body to another, or from a donor to a patient

vaccines medicines that prevent disease

X-rays type of radiation, useful in medicine because they pass through flesh but not bone, allowing doctors to 'see' broken bones

INDEX

A
alchemists 38
alcohol 61, 88–9, 101
almshouses 40
amputations 22, 60–1, 116, 126
amulet 46
anaesthetics 9, 22, 61–3
anatomy 8, 11, 15, 42–3
antibiotics 9, 55, 83–5, 97
antiseptics 9, 64–5, 108, 126
apothecaries 22
arsenic 96
aseptic surgery 67, 108, 126
  see also surgery
astrology 16, 18

B
bacteria 9, 57, 82–3
bad air 8–9, 16, 18, 25, 36, 46, 54–5, 75–6
barber surgeons 18, 22
Bazalgette, Joseph 79
Bevan, Aneurin 94
Beveridge, William 9, 94
Beveridge Report 1942 9
Black Death 1348–49 8, 24–5
blood circulation 42–3
blood groups 98, 109
bloodletting 8, 15, 18, 36
blood transfusions 9, 98, 109, 128–9
Broad Street pump 75–6

C
cancer 98, 102–3
capillaries 43
carbolic acid 64–5
Casualty Clearing Stations (CCS) 118, 119, 123
cesspools 74, 76
Chadwick, Edwin 77
Chain, Ernst 84–5
chemical cures 38, 55
chemical drugs 83, 96
  see also antibiotics
chemotherapy 98, 103
chloroform 62–3
cholera epidemic 1848–49 74–6
Church, role of 11, 14–15, 17, 20, 27
circulation 42–3
Covid-19 pandemic 101
Crick, Francis 87
Culpepper, Nicholas 37
cure-alls 37, 66
Curie, Marie 98

D
Davy, Humphrey 61
diagnosis, modern Britain 90–1
disease
  causes of 8–9, 16, 24–5, 30–5, 46, 54–7
  prevention 8–9, 18, 25, 36, 48, 70–7, 100–2
  treatment 8–9, 17–22, 25, 36–8, 47, 58, 66–9, 83–9, 98–9
dissection 14–15, 21–2, 30, 43
Divine Right 17
DNA (deoxyribonucleic acid) 9, 86–7

E
Ehrlich, Paul 96
ether 61, 63

F
First Aid Nursing Yeomanry (FANY) 121
First World War 1914–18 see Western Front 1914–18
Fleming, Alexander 82–3
Florey, Howard 84–5
Four Humours 8, 14–16, 18, 25
free school meals 93

G
Galen, Claudius 8, 11, 14–15, 22, 42–3
gangrene 64, 119, 126
genes 9, 86
Germ Theory 9, 54–6, 71–2, 79
God, beliefs about disease 8, 16–17, 25, 33, 46
government and public health 9, 11, 48, 71, 76–9, 92–5, 101
Great Fire of London 1666 48
Great Plague 1665 33, 46–8
Gutenberg, Johannes 35

H
Harvey, William 8, 11, 42–3
herbal remedies 8–9, 19, 25, 36–7, 47
Hippocrates 8, 15
hospitals 8, 20, 40, 58, 66, 95, 98, 123
Human Genome Project 87
humours see Four Humours

I
Industrial Revolution 9, 74
infection 20, 58, 63–5, 119, 126
inoculation 70

J
Jenner, Edward 9, 70–1

K
keyhole surgery 99
Koch, Robert 54–5, 57, 65, 83, 96

L
Landsteiner, Karl 98, 109
laughing gas 61
leprosy 20
life expectancy 10, 92
lifestyle 18, 88–9, 101
ligatures 108
Listen, Robert 61
Lister, Joseph 64–5, 83, 108
Lloyd George, David 93
lung cancer 102–3

M
magic bullets 83, 96
Miasma Theory 8–9, 16, 18, 25, 36, 46, 54–5, 75–6
microbes 33
microorganisms 33, 35
midwifery 22, 62
monarchy, role of 17, 38

N
National Health Service (NHS) 9, 11, 94–5
National Insurance Act 1911 93
Nightingale, Florence 58–9
nitrous oxide 61, 63
No Man's Land 112
nursing 59, 121

P
Pasteur, Louis 9, 54–5, 64–5, 72–3, 79, 83
pasteurisation 54
penicillin 82–4, 97
pest houses 41
physicians 8, 21–2, 41
plague 8, 24–5, 33, 46–8
plastic surgery 99, 128
poison gas 118
pollution 77–8
poverty 92–3
prayer 8, 17, 25
printing press 35, 37
PTSD (Post Traumatic Stress Disorder) 117
public health see government and public health
Public Health Act 1875 77–9
purging 8, 18, 36

Q
Queen Alexandra's Imperial Military Nursing Service (QAIMNS) 121

R
radiation therapy 98, 103
Regimental Aid Posts (RAPs) 122
Renaissance 11, 32
Röntgen, Wilhelm 98, 109
Royal Army Medical Corps (RAMC) 116–19, 120, 123–4
Royal Society 8, 35

S
sanitation 76–9
Second World War 1939–45 94
shell shock 112, 117
Simpson, James 62
smallpox 41, 70–1
smoking 37, 74, 88–9, 101, 102
Snow, John 75–6, 77–8
spontaneous generation 55, 56
superstition 22, 38
surgery 9, 55, 60–5, 67, 99, 103, 108, 126–8
Sydenham, Thomas 8, 34
syphilis 96

T
Thomas, Hugh Owen 127
tobacco 37
transference 38
transplants 99
trench fever 116
trench foot 116

V
vaccinations 9, 54, 57, 71–3, 100–1
Vesalius, Andreas 8, 11, 30

W
war and conflict 9, 58–9, 82, 84–5, 94, 110
Watson, James 87
weapons, injuries from 118–19
Western Front 1914–18
  common illnesses 116
  trench life 112–13, 116–17
  wounds and the wounded 114, 118–19, 122–4, 126–9

X
X-rays 109, 127–8